Frontiers in HIV Research
(*Volume 1*)
Advances in HIV Treatment
HIV Enzyme Inhibitors and Antiretroviral Therapy

Edited By

Gene D. Morse

New York State Center of Excellence in Bioinformatics and Life Sciences
University at Buffalo (UB)
Buffalo, New York
USA

&

Sarah Nanzigu

Department of Pharmacology and Therapeutics
Makerere University College of Health Science
Kampala
Uganda

CONTENTS

FOREWORD

It is over three decades since man started battling the human immunodeficiency virus and the diseases associated with it. Although HIV has caused millions of deaths especially in Sub-Saharan Africa, no fully reliable cure or prevention of the viral transmission has been identified. Drugs that suppress viral replication (antiretrovirals) remain the only hope for millions of persons infected with the virus. Since the approval of the first antiretroviral agent in 1985, over 30 such products have been registered. Treatment regimens changed from single drug therapies to combinations with highly active antiretroviral drugs, and those combinations also keep changing with new information and therapies. Consolidated updates on data and evidence of effectiveness of these drugs need to be availed to scientists and clinical practitioners. The ever increasing information motivated the writing of a comprehensive book containing consolidated information on the different available and upcoming antiretroviral agents. This book, edited by Prof. Gene Morse and Dr. Sarah Nanzigu provides these materials with considerations of approaches by experts from developed and developing settings. We highly appreciate these experts for their valued input.

This book with updated information on therapies used in HIV management is carefully relayed under respective classes of drugs including Reverse Transcriptase Inhibitors (RTIs), Protease Inhibitors (PI), Integrase Strand Inhibitors (INSTI), and Entry Inhibitors. Clinically relevant information regarding activity of these agents in different populations is also presented, including comparison of treatment options between resource-limited and resource-rich settings, together with its implications. The book is carefully constructed to become a very valuable asset for scientists and clinicians at different levels of understanding of these drugs. We will highly appreciate feedback from our esteemed readers.

Charles Chiedza Maponga
School of Pharmacy
College of Health Sciences
University of Zimbabwe
Avondale, Harare
Zimbabwe

PREFACE

This book focuses on updates in HIV Treatments, an area with a very high turnover of information. Although there aren't as many new findings related to the human immunodeficiency virus itself, the number of new drugs and targets has grown tremendously since the onset of the epidemic. Treatment guidelines are revised much more often than those of other diseases in order to capture new therapies, changes in regimens, including their indications.

Since the onset of HIV epidemic, more than 30 antiretroviral agents have been approved for use in persons infected with the virus, and those at high risk. Although these drugs are grouped in less than 6 classes, each of them possesses some unique characteristics. These unique attributes can influence vital areas including response to treatment and toxicity profiles. This book is intended to provide compiled and updated information on each of the available and upcoming antiretroviral agents, to assist persons involved in HIV clinical care and research.

The authors have been selected based on their expertise in HIV/AIDS, and we greatly appreciate your valued input into this work. We trust that our esteemed readers will find this information to be of great value.

Gene D. Morse
New York State Center of Excellence in Bioinformatics and Life Sciences
University at Buffalo (UB),
Buffalo, New York
USA

&

Sarah Nanzigu
Department of Pharmacology and Therapeutics
Makerere University College of Health Science
Kampala
Uganda

CONTRIBUTORS

Amy Moss — Thomas Street Health Center, Harris Health System, Houston, TX, USA

Cara Felton — School of Pharmacy and Pharmaceutical Sciences, University at Buffalo, Buffalo, NY, USA

Charles S. Venuto — Translational Pharmacology Research Core, New York State Center of Excellence in Bioinformatics and Life Sciences; School of Pharmacy and Pharmaceutical Sciences, University at Buffalo, Buffalo, NY, USA

Cindy J. Bednasz — Translational Pharmacology Research Core, New York State Center of Excellence in Bioinformatics and Life Sciences; School of Pharmacy and Pharmaceutical Sciences, University at Buffalo, Buffalo, NY, USA

Francis Xavier Kasujja — Médecins Sans Frontières, Harare, Zimbabwe

Gene D. Morse — Translational Pharmacology Research Core, New York State Center of Excellence in Bioinformatics and Life Sciences; School of Pharmacy and Pharmaceutical Sciences, University at Buffalo, Buffalo, NY, USA; Center for Human Experimental Therapeutics, University of Rochester, Rochester NY, USA

Immaculate Nankya — Joint Clinic Research Centre; Kampala,Uganda

Jaran Eriksen — Department of Laboratory Medicine, Division of Clinical Pharmacology, University Hospital at Huddinge, Karolinska Institutet, Sweden

Joshua R. Sawyer — Translational Pharmacology Research Core, New York State Center of Excellence in Bioinformatics and Life Sciences; School of Pharmacy and Pharmaceutical Sciences, University at Buffalo, NY, USA; Erie County Medical Center Corporation, Buffalo, NY, USA

Kevin Hsu — School of Pharmacy and Pharmaceutical Sciences, University at Buffalo, Buffalo, NY, USA

Moses R. Kamya — School of Medicine, Makerere University College of Health Sciences, Uganda

Pauline Byakika Kibwika — Department of Medicine, College of Health Sciences, Makerere University, Uganda

Qing Ma — Translational Pharmacology Research Core, New York State Center of Excellence in Bioinformatics and Life Sciences; School of Pharmacy and Pharmaceutical Sciences, University at Buffalo, Buffalo, NY, USA

Rebecca A. Sumner — Translational Pharmacology Research Core, New York State Center of Excellence in Bioinformatics and Life Sciences; School of Pharmacy and Pharmaceutical Sciences, University at Buffalo, Buffalo, NY, USA; Erie County Medical Center Corporation, Buffalo, NY, USA

Sarah Nanzigu — Department of Pharmacology and Therapeutics, Makerere University College of Health Science, Kampala, Uganda

ACKNOWLEDGEMENTS

The editors and authors would like to appreciate the following people for their various contributions during the writing of this book. They may not have contributed to the actual writing of book chapters, but their availability to; coordinate, guide or counsel was of great benefit to the making of this project.

We appreciate Dr. Michael Makanga, Director South-South, European & Developing Countries Clinical Trials Partnership (EDCTP), for the guidance and encouragement offered at several stages of this writing. We appreciate that you kept open doors for consultations.

The editors and authors would like to acknowledge the coordinating activities rendered by Mrs. Farzia S. Kaufman, Senior Health Information Research Support Specialist Translational Pharmacology Research Core, NYS Center of Excellence in Bioinformatics and Life Sciences, University at Buffalo. Without you, this piece of work could not have been a success.

Appreciation further goes to Mr. Davis Odero Osiemo of Odero Osiemo and Company Advocates, Nairobi, Kenya. The guidance and counsel obtained from your expertise was of great help.

2

CHAPTER 1

Introduction

Sarah Nanzigu[1,*], Francis Xavier Kasujja[2] and Immaculate Nankya[3]

[1]Department of Pharmacology and Therapeutics, Makerere University College of Health Sciences, Kampala, Uganda; [2]Médecins Sans Frontières, Harare-Zimbabwe and [3]Joint Clinical Research Center, Kampala, Uganda

Abstract: Over thirty antiretroviral agents have been developed since the beginning of the fight against the human immunodeficiency virus (HIV). This breakthrough was fostered by the enormous leaps made in understanding viral replication, a cycle that begins with the interaction between the virus and the host cell, usually a CD4-bearing T-lymphocyte. This results into the fusion of the viral membrane with the cellular plasma membrane and the transfer of viral material, including RNA, into the cytoplasm of the host cell. Then, using viral DNA-dependent RNA reverse transcriptase, viral DNA is formed from RNA. Viral DNA is soon translocated to the host cell nucleus where it is integrated into the host DNA in a reaction catalyzed by integrase enzyme. The proviral DNA formed at this stage is used to produce immature viral polypeptides that are eventually cleaved and packaged into mature virions by protease enzyme. Drugs have been developed that target each of these steps; they include entry inhibitors, reverse transcriptase inhibitors, integrase inhibitors, and protease inhibitors. The reverse transcriptase inhibitor, Zidovudine, a nucleoside analogue, was the first antiretroviral agent to be approved in 1987. It was followed by many other nucleotide, nucleoside and non-nucleoside reverse transcriptase inhibitors, and eventually, by protease inhibitors, integrase inhibitors and entry inhibitors. Other viral targets are still under research.

Keywords: HIV drugs, HIV Treatment, Antiretroviral drugs, Antiretroviral therapy, Retroviral treatment, Reverse transcriptase inhibitors, Protease inhibitors, Integrase inhibitors, HIV entry inhibitors, HIV vaccines, ART.

BACKGROUND

For over three decades, man has been battling human immunodeficiency virus (HIV), the infection that leads to acquired immunodeficiency syndrome (AIDS). With time, the infection, its signs, as well as its symptoms have been defined. A deeper understanding of the viral reproductive cycle has fostered the discovery of a number of potential drug targets. To date, over 30 therapeutic agents have been approved for use against HIV infection in humans.

*Corresponding author Sarah Nanzigu: Department of Pharmacology and Therapeutics, Makerere University College of Health Sciences, Kampala, Uganda; Tel: 256784843045; Fax: 256414532947; E-mails: snanzigu@yahoo.com; snanzigu@chs.mak.ac.ug

HIV Case Definition

The initial HIV/AIDS case definition was first built on the occurrence of a rare opportunistic infection (OI), pneumocystis carinii pneumonia (PCP), among previously healthy homosexual young men in Los Angeles [1, 2]. The Centers for Disease Control and Prevention (CDC) and World Health Organization (WHO) case definitions have since evolved to include both the case definition used in HIV infection surveillance and the infection's clinical classification [3].

Criteria for the Diagnosis of HIV Infection

To confirm HIV infection, either laboratory or clinical evidence is required. Laboratory evidence is the more preferred of the two criteria. The 2014 revised case definition for persons aged ≥18 months and children aged <18 months whose mothers were not infected prior to their birth constitutes the following [3]:

- ***Laboratory Evidence**:* HIV positive results, obtained from multitest algorithms – an initial HIV antibody or antigen test and an orthogonal validation test – or stand-alone virological tests. Stand-alone virological or non-antibody tests (NAT) includes qualitative HIV DNA/RNA tests, quantitative HIV viral load assays, the HIV-1 p24 antigen test, HIV isolation (viral culture) and nucleotide sequence (genotype) tests [3].

- ***Clinical Evidence**:* The clinical criteria for HIV case definition are used when surveillance laboratory evidence is unavailable or otherwise inadequate. The criteria are met by the presence of a note in the patient's medical records (made by a physician or other qualified medical-care providers) stating that the individual has HIV infection, and at least one of the following conditions:

  o Laboratory criteria based on tests done after the physician's note was written (validating the note retrospectively).

  o Presumptive evidence of HIV infection (for instance, through receipt of HIV antiretroviral therapy or prophylaxis for an opportunistic infection, an otherwise unexplained low CD4+ T-lymphocyte count, or an otherwise unexplained diagnosis of an opportunistic illness).

For the purpose of surveillance, a confirmed case of HIV infection can be classified into one of five HIV infection stages (0, 1, 2, 3, or unknown) based on the criteria shown in Table **1** [3].

Table 1. Revised HIV case surveillance staging based on CD4 T-lymphocytes.

Stage	Age (in years) at CD4 testing					
	<1		1-5		>6	
	CD4 Cells/μL	CD4 Cell %	CD4 Cells/μL	CD4 Cell %	CD4 Cells/μL	CD4 Cell %
0 early HIV infection	Negative or indeterminate HIV result within 180 days of a confirmed positive result					
1	≥1,500	≥34	≥1,000	≥30	≥500	≥26
2	750–1,499	26–33	500–999	22–29	200–499	14–25
3*	<750	<26	<500	<22	<200	<14
Unknown	no information on CD4+ T-lymphocyte count or percentage					

CD4-T-lymphocyte counts should preferably be used in staging but percentages may be used if cell counts are not available [3].
*In the presence of stage 3–defining opportunistic infections, the staging is 3 regardless of CD4 T-lymphocyte results, except if the criteria for stage 0 are met

THE PATHOGENESIS, MORBIDITY AND MORTALITY IN HIV

HIV attacks the immune system, predominantly destroying T-Lymphocytes in the process. This causes a progressive deterioration in immunity that leads to acquired immunodeficiency syndrome (AIDS). The poor immunity attracts different opportunistic infections and cancers, causing a high morbidity and mortality among HIV-infected persons. At least 20 opportunistic illnesses/ conditions have been described in HIV/AIDS patients. These are listed below (Table **2**) according to their relationship with the progressive decline in CD4 T-lymphocytes [4].

Table 2. Opportunistic infections observed during the course of HIV/AIDS.

>500	200-500	100-200	50-100	<50
- Low risk of OIs - Vaginal Candidiasis or other minor infections	- Candidiasis - Kaposi's sarcoma	- Pneumocystis Jirovecii (Carinii) Pneumonia (PCP) - Histoplasmosis - Coccidioidomycosis - Progressive Multifocal Leukoencephalopathy (PML)	- Toxoplasmosis - Cryptosporidiosis - Cryptococcosis - Cytomegalovirus (CMV)	Mycobacterium Avium Complex (MAC)

Common Causes of Mortality and Morbidity Among HIV/AIDS Patients.

Prior to the era of universal access to ART, AIDS-related conditions (AR) (as listed in Table **2**) [5-11] were the leading cause of morbidity and mortality among HIV-infected patients globally. However, access to ART has improved markedly, altering the epidemiologic picture in some low and middle income countries to mirror the morbidity and mortality trends in the more equitable high income countries where non-AIDS related conditions, such as non-AIDS related cancers (NAC), are now the leading cause of death [12-15]. Even then, AIDS-related conditions including cancers, still drive morbidity and mortality in sub-Saharan Africa and some parts of Europe and Asia [12, 13, 16, 17]. Besides, Tuberculosis remains the leading cause of death both in the pre-universal and universal era of ART access [5, 12, 17, 18].

HIV MOLECULAR STRUCTURE

HIV was first described by Barre-Sinossi *et al.*, in 1983 as a T-lymphotropic retrovirus following its initial isolation from a Caucasian patient presenting with signs and symptoms characteristics of AIDS [19]. It is a retrovirus in the Lentiviridae sub-family that carries its genetic material in the form of ribonucleic acid (RNA) rather than de-oxyribonucleic acid (DNA) [20, 21]. Retroviruses use the reverse transcriptase enzyme to synthesize a DNA molecule complementary to the RNA template. Under the electronic microscope, HIV appears as spherical particles, called virions, each containing two RNA strands enclosed within a nuclear capsid [20, 22] (Fig. **1**). Enclosed together with the RNA strands are the enzymes required for viral replication: reverse transcriptase, integrase and protease. Each virion is covered with a fatty coat, the viral envelope, bearing several projections made up of glycoproteins, gp120 and gp41[23]. These glycoproteins are non-covalently associated units, formed after the glycosylation and cleavage of their precursor, gp160. The gp120 subunit remains as an envelope glycoprotein while gp41 is a trans-membrane subunit [23]. The former (gp120) is made up of 5 conserved regions (C1-C5), the main areas of contact with gp41, and 5 variable regions/loops (V1-V5), which serve specific roles. V1, V2 and V3 shield the conserved regions from antibody recognition [24]; the V3 loop additionally determines viral tropism [23, 25, 26]. The gp41 subunit consists of an amino-terminal (N) peptide and a carboxy-terminal (C), and the subunit is believed to exist in two major conformational states: the native or non-fusogenic state and the fusion-active state [23, 25].

The virus has nine genes, three of which, namely; *gag*, *pol* and *env*, code for viral replication. The other six – *tat*, *rev*, *nef*, *vif*, *vpr* and *vpu* – code for the proteins necessary for the infective process.

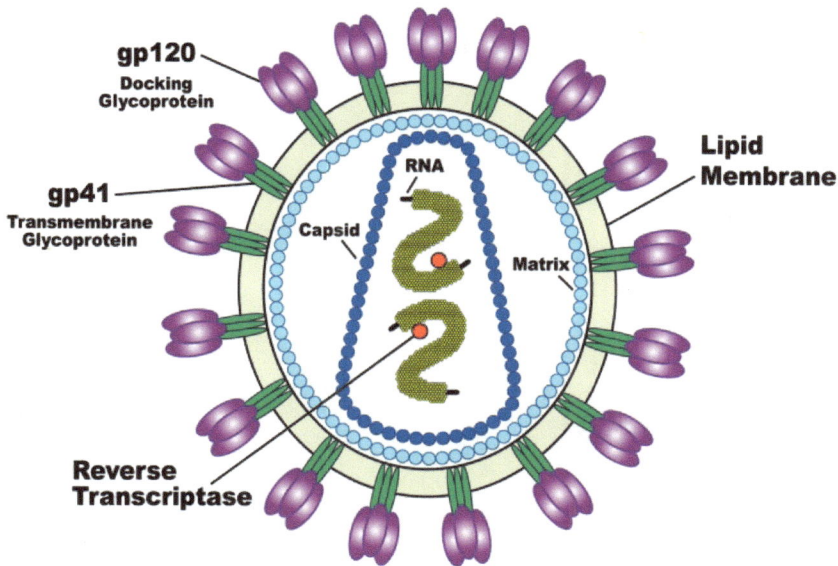

http://en.wikipedia.org/wiki/Structure_and_genome_of_HIV#mediaviewer/File:HIV_Virion-en-2.png

Fig. (1). Simplified diagram of the human immunodeficiency virus (HIV) [22, 27].

THE MOLECULAR STRUCTURE AND ROLE OF THE HOST CELL

The Helper T-lymphocyte – a T-cell subset that bears CD4 molecules and recognizes antigens associated with class II Major Histocompatibility Cells (MHC) – is the primary target of HIV [28-30]. Monocytes, neutrophils, eosinophils and tissue macrophages, are some of the other targets of the virus, however, a more aggressive and cytopathological infection is observed in T-Lymphocyte leading to progressive immunosuppression [31-34].

The CD4 terminology signifies a cluster of differentiation (CD) destined for the T cell antigen "T4/leu3" [35]. CD4 molecules are 55kd and are found on the surface of the subset of T-lymphocytes (Fig. **2**), and the molecules act as HIV receptors on the cell membranes of the targeted cells [21-23, 29, 30].

CD4 T-lymphocytes also have chemokine receptors that act as co-receptors during HIV infection. At least 19 of these chemokine receptors have been described and are grouped into 4 sub-families: CXC chemokine receptors (CXCR1 to CXCR6), CC chemokine receptors (CCR1 to CCR10), CX_3C chemokine receptors (only CX_3CR1) and XC chemokine receptors (only XCR1)[36]. A fifth sub-family, ACK is still under review but ACKR3 co-receptor is already described under the sub-family [36].

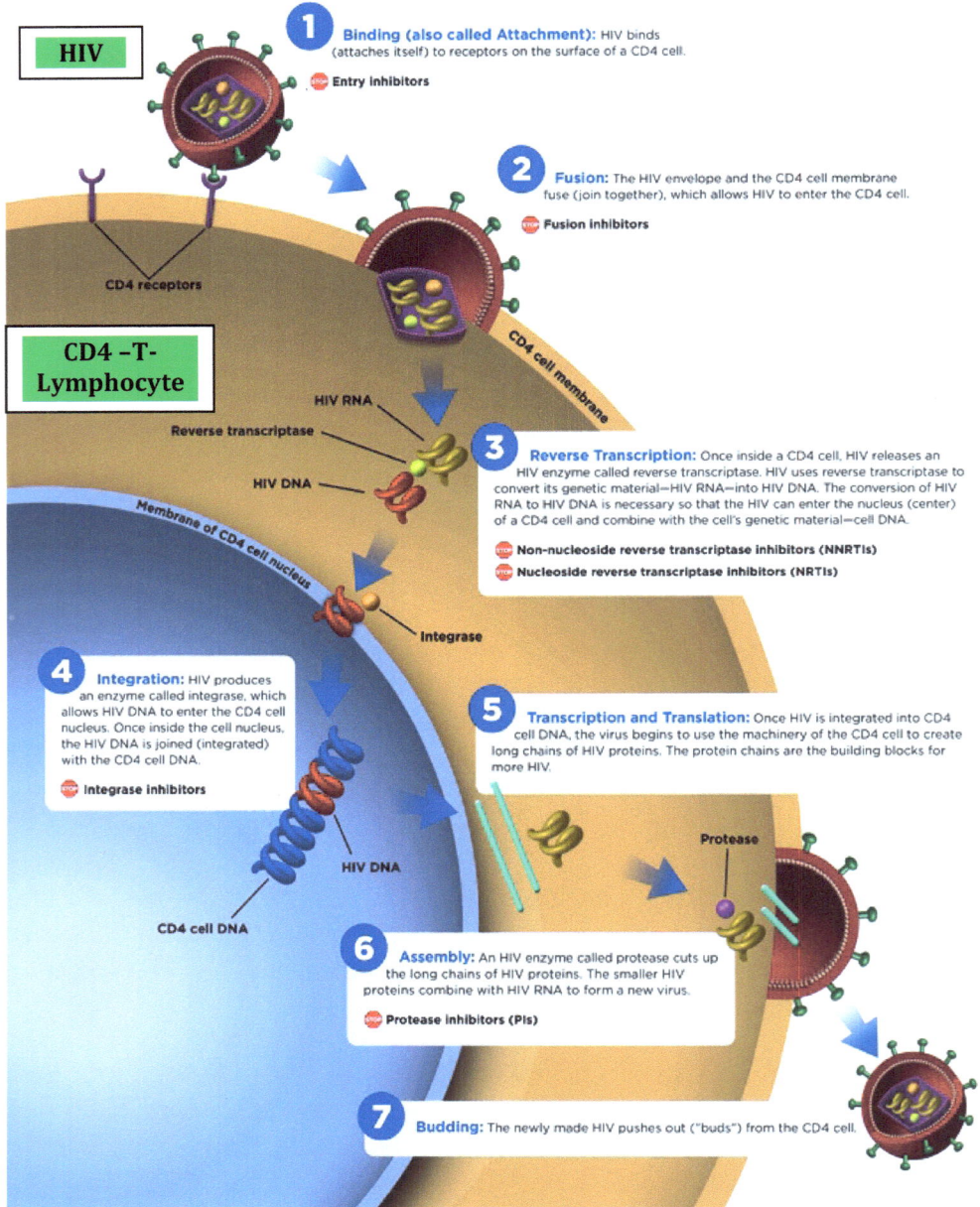

Fig. (2). Illustration of HIV replication cycle and the drug targets [133].

CCR5 and CXCR4 are the main HIV 1 and HIV 2 co-receptors [37-39]. CCR5 co-receptor, also known as CD195 or the macrophage-tropic (M-Tropic) co-receptor predominates during early infection while the T-cell line tropic (T-tropic) CXCR4 co-receptor comes into play during later stages of the infection [38, 40]. Minor CD4 co-receptors, including CCR2, detected on human CD4 T-lymphocytes and monocytes [41, 42], and CCR3, on CNS microglia cells [40, 41], act as HIV co-receptors to varying extents [43-45]. Information on the role of CCR6, CXCR3, and CXCR5 in HIV co-reception is limited [46-49].

HIV AND THE HOST-CELL INTERACTIONS

At the beginning of the HIV infection process, the viral envelop glycoprotein, gp120, binds to the CD4 cell receptor (Fig. **2**), exposing the V3 loop and enabling them to bind to the CCR5/CXCR4 co-receptors of the host cell [50-52]. The configuration of the variable region of the env glycoprotein, the V3 loop, determines the viral co-receptor tropism [23]: macrophage-tropic viruses that predominate in the initial stages of the infection use the CCR5 co-receptor and, to a lesser extent, CCR3 receptor [40, 53, 54]; on the contrary, T-cell-line-tropic (T-tropic) viruses attach to CXCR4 co-receptors [40, 55].

The attachment of the HIV virus to the CD4 receptor and the co-receptor triggers a conformational change in the gp41 to expose its fusion peptide, heralding a shift to a fusion-active state that facilitates viral fusion to the CD4 host cell [23, 25] (Fig. **2**). These conformational changes are slow reactions, believed to be initiated within 1-4 minutes of receptor/co-receptor attachment and completed within 20 minutes. A stable fusion-active conformation state is then reached [23]. The slow intermediate state gives room for attack with specific antiretroviral agents.

After the fusion of the virus with the host cell membrane, HIV releases its genetic material and enzymes into the host cell. This marks the beginning of the replication process. The first step in this process involves the formation of viral DNA from RNA using the reverse transcriptase enzyme. The newly formed viral DNA consists of a long terminal repeat sequence of GT and AC nucleotides at both the 3' and 5' ends [56, 57]. It is necessary for Viral DNA to be translocated into the host nucleus in order for it to be incorporated into the host DNA. To this end viral integrase, acting within the host cell cytoplasm cleaves the GT dinucleotide from the 3' end (3' processing), creating a reactive hydroxyl group of the CA dinucleotide, at that end, that attacks the host DNA [58-60]. Integrase further catalyzes viral DNA strand transfer into host DNA by activating host DNA attack by the reactive hydroxyl group [61].

The HIV integrase enzyme comprises of 3 domains including the catalytic core domain (CCD) that contains the enzyme's active site [62, 63]. The catalytic domain has three amino acids (D64, D116 and E152) that bind the divalent metals – either Mg^{2+} or Mn^{2+} [60, 64-66] – to coordinate the bonding of the enzyme with viral DNA during 3' processing and strand transfer. Integration culminates in the formation of proviral DNA.

Once integrated into host DNA, the provirus can now be used to replicate and form new viral components: long polypeptides, consisting of viral RNA, and core enzymes. The viral components gather at the cell membrane of the host cell where immature viruses bud off (Fig. **2**) and are cut into smaller functional proteins (mature virions) by the protease enzyme [67]. These then proceed to infect other host cells.

PHARMACOLOGICAL AGENTS TARGETING HIV REPLICATION

A significant amount of research has gone into exploring the HIV replication cycle in search of potential therapeutic interventions [68]. This has led to the discovery of a wide selection of antiretroviral agents, mainly inhibitors against the viral processes; entry, reverse transcription, viral cleavage. The available agents are listed in appendix **1** of this chapter. Research in the novel areas of maturation inhibitors and immune simulation gene therapy is also gaining ground.

Agents Targeting HIV Entry Process

These agents belong to one of the following three groups:

1. Inhibitors of the interaction between the viral surface glycoprotein gp120 and the CD4 molecule,

2. Inhibitors of the interaction between gp120 and CCR5 or CXCR4

3. (Chemokines and related agents that antagonize chemokine receptor activity) [69].

    i. The CCR5-receptor blocker, Maraviroc is an example (appendix 1). Research for selective CXCR4-receptor antagonists is ongoing [70].

    ii. Given the ability of HIV to have dual receptor utilization, research for non-selective chemokine receptor antagonists is ongoing. Cenicriviroc, a CCR5/CCR2 antagonist, showed promising results from Phase II trials [71-73].

4. Fusion inhibitors. These are peptides derived from the sequence of the viral trans-membrane glycoprotein gp41), including synthetic C-peptides and or N-peptides that inhibit transition of the gp41 to its fusion-active conformation state [74-76]. Enfuvirtide (T20) is an HIV-1 gp41 C-terminal peptide derivative [76]. One of the advantages of this agent is its activity against HIV strains that utilize the CCR5, CXCR4 co-receptors, and the dual-tropic strains that utilize both co-receptors [77, 78].

Experimental agents include dual co-receptor antagonists [71-73]; monoclonal antibodies, including PRO 140, which contains genetically-engineered antibodies that bind to the CCR5 co-receptor [79, 80], and an anti-CD4 monoclonal antibody, Ibalizumab (TMB-355), which binds to, and blocks, the T-cell CD4 receptor [81].

Agents Targeting the Reverse Transcription Step

The step during which the viral DNA is synthesized from RNA by the DNA-dependent RNA reverse transcriptase enzyme can be inhibited by agents belonging to the following categories:

1. Nucleoside reverse transcriptase inhibitors (NRTI). These are nucleoside analogues that compete for, and block, the reverse transcriptase enzyme [82]. Zidovudine was the first NRTI to be approved in 1987 [83, 84]. Since then, several others agents have been approved by the Food and Drug Act (FDA), including Didanosine, Abacavir and Lamivudine [84-88] (see appendix 1).

2. Nucleotide reverse transcriptase inhibitors (NtRTI). These are nucleotide analogues that compete for and block the reverse transcriptase enzyme. Tenofovir, an adenosine monophosphate analogue, is an example [89, 90].

3. Non-nucleoside reverse transcriptase inhibitors (NNRTI). These agents are not analogues of the natural DNA bases. They bind to a secondary allosteric site far from the active site of the reverse transcriptase enzyme. This causes a stereochemical change in the

enzyme that reduces its affinity to naturally-occurring nucleosides [91, 92]. In this way, the addition of new nucleotides to the growing viral DNA chain is hindered. Approved agents in this category include Efavirenz, Nevirapine, Delavirdine, Etravirine, and Rilpivirine [91].

Agents Targeting the Integration Process

Viral DNA integration can be inhibited at several stages; however, known pharmacologically-active agents target the integrase enzyme during 3' processing and viral DNA strand transfer. All the currently registered integrase inhibitors target the strand transfer process, and research on agents active against 3' processing is ongoing.

1. Agents that block Viral DNA strand transfer

    These agents compete with the HIV DNA substrate for the integrase enzyme; some agents may chelate the Mg^{2+}/Mn^{2+} metals ions in the CCD domain [61]. The diketoacid derivative Raltegravir was the first FDA registered integrase strand inhibitor. It was soon followed by Elvitegravir and Dolutegravir [93].

2. Agents that inhibit both 3' processing and strand transfer

    These agents are still undergoing research; they include both Strylquinolone and Phenyldipyrimidine derivatives [61, 94].

Agents Targeting the Action of Protease Enzyme

Protease inhibitors bind to the site where protein-cutting occurs, preventing the enzyme from releasing mature virions [95]. Several agents in this category have been registered.

1. Agents Active against HIV-1 Protease Enzyme,

    These include: Indinavir, Nelfinavir, Ritonavir, Amprenavir, Atazanavir, [96-98].

2. Agents Active against Both HIV-1 and HIV-2 Protease Enzymes

    These include: Lopinavir, Saquinavir, Tipranavir, and Darunavir [96-98].

Other Emerging Targets of Antiretroviral Agents

Other emerging targets of antiretroviral agents include maturation inhibitors. These prevent late-stage gag polyprotein-processing but are not active against the protease enzyme. Bevirimat is an example of this drug category [68, 99]. Immune stimulation and gene therapy is another emerging category [99].

RNA-based Therapies

RNA-based immunotherapy approaches and prophylactic vaccines against HIV-associated cancers and infectious diseases are under investigation; specifically, microRNAs (miRNAs) are being explored for their potential use against HIV. While conventional large RNA families (including mRNA, tRNA and rRNA) convey and translate genetic information from DNA into proteins during the synthesis of the latter, miRNAs in contrast, are small non-coding RNAs, that mainly serve as post-transcriptional regulators of gene expression [100-104]. They are partially complementary to sequences in mRNA, and binding of miRNAs to complementary sites on target mRNAs may down regulate productive translation or induce cleavage thus accelerating mRNA degradation [104]. Cellular miRNAs are important in modulation of cellular susceptibility, and the replication and virulence of HIV-1. They have been shown to play a role in HIV non progressors, through their ability to suppress HIV Nef, a protein known to mediate immune evasion by HIV [105-110]. This has made both miRNAs and the Nef protein potential targets in the search for additional HIV therapies.

Unlike RNA viruses, several DNA viruses encode for functional miRNAs [111]. Retroviruses, on the other hand, have access to both nuclear and cytoplasmic miRNA processing machinery, and have been shown to express functional miRNAs. The bovine leukemia retrovirus, for example, has been shown to encode an RNA pol III-transcribed miRNA cluster and computational algorithms predict that HIV-1 can encode five candidate viral miRNAs [111, 112]. Studies have demonstrated the presence of functional miRNAs within the HIV-1 RNA genome including the Nef-U3-miR-N367 in the HIV-1 Nef coding region; the HIV-1-miR-H1 at the 3′ end of the HIV-1 RNA; and TAR-miR-5p and 3p at the HIV-1 transactivation RNA (TAR). Certain anti-HIV-1 miRNAs that are highly expressed in resting $CD4^+$ T cells – miR-28, miR-125b, miR-150, miR-223, and miR-382 – are able to bind to the HIV-1 RNA and inhibit HIV-1 infection [113]. Besides, research has demonstrated that overexpression of miRNAs may interfere with the RNA-Gag interaction through formation of miRNA-Gag complexes. This leads to the blocking of HIV-1 viral budding at the plasma membrane of the host cell hence reducing viral infectivity.

HIV Vaccine Research

Although no HIV vaccine has yet been approved by the FDA, several candidates are undergoing trial. These include prophylactic vaccines – comprising the vast majority of the candidates – aimed at HIV prevention, and vaccines that delay disease progression to AIDS among HIV-infected persons. Preventive vaccines generally elicit the production of neutralizing antibodies (Nabs) that target gp120 of the env protein; while T-cell vaccines reduce viral replication after infection thereby slowing and/or reducing transmission of HIV from the infected persons [24, 114, 115]. Most clinical trials have involved preventive vaccines.

Vaccine success is hampered by several factors: the virus's propensity for mutation and host immune evasion. The extensive viral subtype and sequence diversity has for long rendered the steps in development of a universal HIV vaccine a highly elusive goal [114, 116]. A successful preventive vaccine should supposedly induce an immune response that can prevent the attachment of the viral env protein gp120 to the host receptor/co-receptor, or it should prevent viral fusion. Nonetheless, the outer face of the gp120 envelope protein is shown to be immunologically silent. The vulnerable exposed regions of the gp120 include the variable regions V1-V5, while the conserved regions are relatively concealed from immune recognition [24, 117]. This gp120 portion can further escape immune recognition by a number of mechanisms, including glycan shielding, mutation of variable regions and conformation masking [118]. Most vaccine candidates target the V1 and V2 loops; those targeting the V3 loop are also under trial although this loop is fairly inaccessible as it is covered by the V1 and V2 loops in some HIV isolates, and anti-V3 loop antibodies are highly strain-specific, limiting the chances of a universal vaccine [118]. To overcome this limitation, current HIV vaccine research has mainly focused on designing candidate vaccines for different populations based on predominating HIV isolates or on designing vaccines that elicit potent and broadly neutralizing antibodies with the ability to block infectivity of a genetically diverse pool of HIV strains [115, 119-121] such as vaccines that target the conserved regions of the env protein [120, 122],

The first two antibody-based vaccines – VAX004, for clade B gp120 and VAX003, for clades B and E gp120 – did not show adequate efficacy; moreover, the first T-cell vaccine, based on the recombinant type 5 adenovirus gag/pol/nef, showed trends towards increased HIV acquisition [123, 124]. After many years of negative vaccine attempts, the RV144phase III trial showed positive results among Thai volunteers who received 4 doses of the prime ALVAC HIV vaccine and 2 booster doses of AIDSVAX B/E vaccine [125]. The vaccine regimen induces T-Cell responses that preferentially target epitopes within the V2 region of HIV-1 envelope [125]. Following the administration of four doses of the ALVAC over a 6-month period, boosted with 2 doses of AIDSVAX B/E at 3 and 6 months, there was a 60% efficacy at 1 year that reduced to 31% after 3.5 years [124, 125]. This vaccine has the potential usage in developing vaccine candidates that express HIV isolates in different regions; the vaccine could also be possibly boosted further to achieve longer-lasting protection [119].

ADDITIONAL ASPECTS REGARDING ANTIRETROVIRAL AGENTS

Resistance emerges very fast during the use of antiretroviral drugs; hence combination rather than monotherapy is the recommended approach. WHO and DHHS Guidelines recommend the of use combinations with drugs from different classes to achieve maximum viral suppression [126, 127]. It should also be noted that there are other factors, including accessibility, drug resistance, variations in HIV types, and host genetic variability, that may influence the choice of antiretroviral agents [128-132].

CONFLICT OF INTEREST

The authors confirm that this chapter contents have no conflict of interest.

ACKNOWLEDGEMENTS

Declared none.

REFERENCES

[1]   Centre for Disease Control (CDC). Pneumocystis pneumonia --- Los Angeles. MMWR 1981; 30:250—2

[2]   CDC. Pneumocystis pneumonia [homepage on the Internet]. Los Angeles: CDC Morbidity and Mortality Weekly Report; [updated: 2nd May 2001; accessed: 21st June 2014]. Available from: http://www.cdc.gov/mmwr/preview/mmwrhtml/june_5.htm/

[3]   Selik RM, Mokotoff ED, Branson B, Michele-Owen SM, Whitmore SM, Hall HI. Morbidity and Mortality: Revised Surveillance Case Definition for HIV Infection — United States. 2014; 63(RR-03): 1-19.

[4]   AIDS.Gov. Opportunistic Infections and Their Relationship to HIV/AIDS [homepage on the Internet]. U.S. Department of Health & Human Services; [update: 16th November 2010: accesses: 24th June 2014]. Available from: http://www.aids.gov/hiv-aids-basics/staying-healthy-with-hiv-aids/potential-related-health-problems/opportunistic-infections/ .

[5]   Bellamy R, Sangeetha S, Paton NI. Causes of death among patients with HIV in Singapore from 1985 to 2001: results from the Singapore HIV Observational Cohort Study (SHOCS). HIV Med 2004; 5(4): 289-95.

[6]   Eskild A, Magnus P, Samuelsen SO, Sohlberg C, Kittelsen P. Differences in mortality rates and causes of death between HIV positive and HIV negative intravenous drug users. Int J Epidemiol 1993; 22(2): 315-20.

[7]   Kravcik S, Hawley-Foss N, Victor G, et al. Causes of death of HIV-infected persons in Ottawa, Ontario, 1984-1995. Arch Intern Med 1997; 157(18): 2069-73.

[8]   Marimoutou C, Poizot-Martin I, Loundou AD, Cassuto JP, Obadia Y, Groupe d'etude M. [Causes of hospitalization and death in the MANIF 2000 cohort, composed of HIV-infected patients contaminated by intravenous drug use, 1995-1999]. Presse Med 2003; 32(13 Pt 1): 587-94.

[9]   Okongo M, Morgan D, Mayanja B, Ross A, Whitworth J. Causes of death in a rural, population-based human immunodeficiency virus type 1 (HIV-1) natural history cohort in Uganda. Int J Epidemiol 1998; 27(4): 698-702.

[10]   Smith DK, Gardner LI, Phelps R, et al. Mortality rates and causes of death in a cohort of HIV-infected and uninfected women, 1993-1999. J Urban Health 2003; 80(4): 676-88.

[11]   Vandentorren S, Mercie P, Marimoutou C, et al. Trends in causes of death in the Aquitaine cohort of HIV-infected patients, 1995-1997. Eur J Epidemiol 2001; 17(1): 7-10.

[12]   Chkhartishvili N, Sharvadze L, Chokoshvili O, et al. Mortality and causes of death among HIV-infected individuals in the country of georgia: 1989-2012. AIDS Res Hum Retroviruses 2014; 30(6): 560-6.

[13]   Ehren K, Hertenstein C, Kummerle T, et al. Causes of death in HIV-infected patients from the Cologne-Bonn cohort. Infection 2014; 42(1): 135-40.

[14]   Fazito E, Vasconcelos AM, Pereira MG, Rezende DF. Trends in non-AIDS-related causes of death among adults with HIV/AIDS, Brazil, 1999 to 2010. Cad Saude Publica 2013; 29(8): 1644-53.

[15]   Ingle SM, May MT, Gill MJ, et al. Impact of Risk Factors for Specific Causes of Death in the First and Subsequent Years of Antiretroviral Therapy Among HIV-Infected Patients. Clin Infect Dis 2014.

[16]   Huang LF, Tang XP, Cai WP, et al. Analysis of death causes of 345 cases with HIV/AIDS in Guangdong area (abstract). Pubmed abstracts 2013; 27(1): 57-60.

[17]   Lewden C, Drabo YJ, Zannou DM, et al. Disease patterns and causes of death of hospitalized HIV-positive adults in West Africa: a multicountry survey in the antiretroviral treatment era. J Int AIDS Soc 2014; 17: 18797.

[18]   Cain KP, Anekthananon T, Burapat C, et al. Causes of death in HIV-infected persons who have tuberculosis, Thailand. Emerg Infect Dis 2009; 15(2): 258-64.

[19]   Barre-Sinoussi F, Chermann JC, Rey F, et al. Isolation of a T-lymphocyte retrovirus from a patient at risk for acquired immunodeficiency syndrome (AIDS). Science 1983; 220: 868-87.

[20]   Avert. HIV Structure and Life Cycle [homepage on the Internet]. Avert [updated: 2010; cited 11 June 2014]. Available from: http: //www.avert.org/hiv-structure-Dand-life-cycle.htm/

[21]   Excellence A. Diagram or Retroviruses [cited: 11June 2014]. Available from: http: //www.accessexcellence.org/RC/VL/GG/diagram.php.

[22]   AVERT. The Structure of HIV. Avert 2010.

[23]   Chan DC, Kim PS. HIV Entry and Its Inhibition. Cell 1998; 93(5): 681-4.

[24]   Pantophlet R, Burton DR. GP120: target for neutralizing HIV-1 antibodies. Annual review of immunology 2006; 24: 739-69.

[25]   Chan DC, Fass D, Berger JM, Kim PS. Core Structure of gp41 from the HIV Envelope Glycoprotein. Cell 1997; 89(2): 263-73.

[26]   Fouchier RA, Groenink M, Kootstra N, et al. Phenotype-associated sequence variation in the third variable domain of the human immunodeficiency virus type 1 gp120 molecule. J Virol 1992 66(5): 3183-7.

[27]   Wekipedia. HIV Virion-en. Weikipedia 2005.

[28]   Dalgleish AG, Beverley PC, Clapham PR, Crawford DH, Greaves MF, Weiss RA. The CD4 (T4) antigen is an essential component of the receptor for the AIDS retrovirus. Nature 1984; 312(5996): 763-7.

[29]   Hoxie JA, Alpers JD, Rackowski JL, *et al.* Alterations in T4 (CD4) protein and mRNA synthesis in cells infected with HIV. Science 1986; 234(4780): 1123-7.

[30]   Lifson JD, Feinberg MB, Reyes GR, *et al.* Induction of CD4-dependent cell fusion by the HTLV-III/LAV envelope glycoprotein. Nature 1986; 323(6090): 725-8.

[31]   Lifson JD, Reyes GR, McGrath MS, Stein BS, Engleman EG. AIDS retrovirus induced cytopathology: giant cell formation and involvement of CD4 antigen. Science 1986; 232(4754): 1123-7.

[32]   Crowe SM. Role of macrophages in the pathogenesis of human immunodeficiency virus (HIV) infection. Aust N Z J Med 1995; 25(6): 777-83.

[33]   Spear GT, Ou CY, Kessler HA, Moore JL, Schochetman G, Landay AL. Analysis of lymphocytes, monocytes, and neutrophils from human immunodeficiency virus (HIV)-infected persons for HIV DNA. J Infect Dis 1990; 162(6): 1239-44.

[34]   Kedzierska K, Crowe SM. The role of monocytes and macrophages in the pathogenesis of HIV-1 infection. Curr Med Chem 2002; 9(21): 1893-903.

[35]   Robey E, Axel R. CD4: collaborator in immune recognition and HIV infection. Cell 1990; 60(5): 697-700.

[36]   Chemokine receptors. [Internet]. IUPHAR database (IUPHAR-DB). 2014 [cited 17/06/2014]. Available from: http: //www.iuphar-db.org/DATABASE/FamilyMenuForward?familyId=14.

[37]   Delezay O, Koch N, Yahi N, Hammache D, Tourres C, Tamalet C, *et al.* Co-expression of CXCR4/fusin and galactosylceramide in the human intestinal epithelial cell line HT-29. Aids 1997; 11(11): 1311-8.

[38]   Albright AV, Shieh JT, Itoh T, *et al.* Microglia express CCR5, CXCR4, and CCR3, but of these, CCR5 is the principal coreceptor for human immunodeficiency virus type 1 dementia isolates. J virol 1999; 73(1): 205-13.

[39]   Chemokine receptors: CCR5 [Internet]. IUPHAR database (IUPHAR-   DB). 2014 [cited 17/06/2014]. Available from: http: //www.iuphar-db.org/DATABASE/ObjectDisplayForward?objectId=62.

[40]   He J, Chen Y, Farzan M, *et al.* CCR3 and CCR5 are co-receptors for HIV-1 infection of microglia. Nature 1997; 385(6617): 645-9.

[41]   Frade JM, Llorente M, Mellado M, *et al.* The amino-terminal domain of the CCR2 chemokine receptor acts as coreceptor for HIV-1 infection. The Journal of clinical investigation 1997; 100(3): 497-502.

[42]   Frade JM, Mellado M, del Real G, Gutierrez-Ramos JC, Lind P, Martinez AC. Characterization of the CCR2 chemokine receptor: functional CCR2 receptor expression in B cells. Journal of immunology 1997; 159(11): 5576-84.

[43]   Lee B, Doranz BJ, Rana S, *et al.* Influence of the CCR2-V64I polymorphism on human immunodeficiency virus type 1 coreceptor activity and on chemokine receptor function of CCR2b, CCR3, CCR5, and CXCR4. J virol 1998; 72(9): 7450-8.

[44]   Rana S, Besson G, Cook DG, *et al.* Role of CCR5 in infection of primary macrophages and lymphocytes by macrophage-tropic strains of human immunodeficiency virus: resistance to patient-derived and prototype isolates resulting from the delta ccr5 mutation. J virol 1997; 71(4): 3219-27.

[45]   Yi Y, Rana S, Turner JD, Gaddis N, Collman RG. CXCR-4 is expressed by primary macrophages and supports CCR5-independent infection by dual-tropic but not T-tropic isolates of human immunodeficiency virus type 1. J virol 1998; 72(1): 772-7.

[46]   Kivisakk P, Trebst C, Lee JC, *et al.* Expression of CCR2, CCR5, and CXCR3 by CD4+ T cells is stable during a 2-year longitudinal study but varies widely between individuals. Journal of neurovirology 2003; 9(3): 291-9.

[47]   Chemokine receptors: CXCR3. [homepage on the Internet]. IUPHAR database (IUPHAR-DB); 2013 [cited   17/06/2014.].   Available   from: http: //www.iuphar-db.org/DATABASE/ObjectDisplayForward?objectId=70.

[48]   Saito R, Onodera H, Tago H, *et al*. Altered expression of chemokine receptor CXCR5 on T cells of myasthenia gravis patients Journal of neuroimmunology 2005; 170(1-2): 172-8.

[49]   Chemokine receptors: CCR6 [Internet]. IUPHAR database (IUPHAR-DB). 2014 [cited 25/06/2014]. Available from: http: //www.iuphar-db.org/DATABASE/ObjectDisplayForward?objectId=63.

[50]   Brand D, Srinivasan K, Sodroski J. Determinants of human immunodeficiency virus type 1 entry in the CDR2 loop of the CD4 glycoprotein. J Virol 1995; 69(1): 166-71.

[51]   Arthos J, Deen KC, Chaikin MA, *et al*. Identification of the residues in human CD4 critical for the binding of HIV. Author information Cell 1989; 57(3): 469-81.

[52]   Chen SS. Functional role of the zipper motif region of human immunodeficiency virus type 1 transmembrane protein gp41. J Virol Mar 1994; 68(3): 2002–2010.; 68(3): 2002–10.

[53]   Alkhatib G, Combadiere C, Broder CC, *et al*. CC CKR5: a RANTES, MIP-1alpha, MIP-1beta receptor as a fusion cofactor for macrophage-tropic HIV-1. Science 1996; 272(5270): 1955-8.

[54]   Choe H, Farzan M, Sun Y, *et al*. The beta-chemokine receptors CCR3 and CCR5 facilitate infection by primary HIV-1 isolates. Cell 1996; 85(7): 1135-48.

[55]   Choe H. Chemokine receptors in HIV-1 and SIV infection. Arch Pharm Res. 1998; 21(6): 634-9.

[56]   Panganiban AT, Temin HM. The retrovirus pol gene encodes a product required for DNA integration: identification of a retrovirus int locus. Proc Natl Acad Sci USA 1984; 81(24): 7885-9.

[57]   Bradley CM, Craigie R. Seeing is believing: structure of the catalytic domain of HIV-1 integrase in complex with human LEDGF/p75. Proc Natl Acad Sci USA 2005; 102(49): 17543-4.

[58]   Guiot E, Carayon K, Delelis O, *et al*. Relationship between the oligomeric status of HIV-1 integrase on DNA and enzymatic activity. J Biol Chem 2006; 281(32): 22707-19.

[59]   Engelman A, Hickman AB, Craigie R. The core and carboxyl-terminal domains of the integrase protein of human immunodeficiency virus type 1 each contribute to nonspecific DNA binding. J Virol 1994; 68(9): 5911-7.

[60]   Esposito D, Craigie R. HIV integrase structure and function. Adv Virus Res 1999; 52: 319-33.

[61]   Craigie R. HIV integrase, a brief overview from chemistry to therapeutics. J Biol Chem 2001; 276(26): 23213-6.

[62]   Engelman A, Bushman FD, Craigie R. Identification of discrete functional domains of HIV-1 integrase and their organization within an active multimeric complex. EMBO J 1993; 12(8): 3269-75.

[63]   Engelman A, Craigie R. Identification of conserved amino acid residues critical for human immunodeficiency virus type 1 integrase function *in vitro*. J Virol 1992; 66(11): 6361-9.

[64]   Goldgur Y, Craigie R, Cohen GH, *et al*. Structure of the HIV-1 integrase catalytic domain complexed with an inhibitor: a platform for antiviral drug design. Proc Natl Acad Sci U S A. 1999; 96(23): 13040-3.

[65]   Goldgur Y, Dyda F, Hickman AB, Jenkins TM, Craigie R, Davies DR. Three new structures of the core domain of HIV-1 integrase: an active site that binds magnesium. Proc Natl Acad Sci USA 1998; 95(16): 9150-4.

[66]   Engelman A, Craigie R. Efficient magnesium-dependent human immunodeficiency virus type 1 integrase activity. J Virol 1995; 69(9): 5908-11.

[67]   Welsch S, Keppler OT, Habermann A, Allespach A, Krijnse-Locker J, Kräusslich H. HIV-1 Buds Predominantly at the Plasma Membrane of Primary Human Macrophages. PLoS Pathog 2007; 3(3).

[68]   Reeves JD, Piefer AJ. Emerging drug targets for antiretroviral therapy. Drugs 2005.

[69]   Heveker N. Chemokine receptors as anti-retroviral targets. Curr Drug Targets 2001; 2(1): 21-39.

[70]   Schols D, Struyf S, Van Damme J, Este JA, Henson G, De Clercq E. Inhibition of T-tropic HIV strains by selective antagonization of the chemokine receptor CXCR4. J Exp Med 1997; 186(8): 1383-8.

[71]   Kagan RM, Johnson EP, Siaw MF, *et al.* Comparison of genotypic and phenotypic HIV type 1 tropism assay: results from the screening samples of Cenicriviroc Study 202, a randomized phase II trial in treatment-naive subjects. AIDS Res Hum Retroviruses 2014; 30(2): 151-9.

[72]   Klibanov OM, Williams SH, Iler CA. Cenicriviroc, an orally active CCR5 antagonist for the potential treatment of HIV infection. Curr Opin Investig Drugs 2010; 11(8): 940-50.

[73]   Menning MM, Dalziel SM. Fumaric acid microenvironment tablet formulation and process development for crystalline cenicriviroc mesylate, a BCS IV compound. Mol Pharm 2013; 10(11): 4005-15.

[74]   Eissmann K, Mueller S, Sticht H, *et al.* HIV-1 fusion is blocked through binding of GB Virus C E2-derived peptides to the HIV-1 gp41 disulfide loop [corrected]. PLoS One 2013; 8(1): e54452.

[75]   Liu S, Zhao Q, Jiang S. Determination of the HIV-1 gp41 fusogenic core conformation modeled by synthetic peptides: applicable for identification of HIV-1 fusion inhibitors. Peptides 2003; 24(9): 1303-13.

[76]   Qi Z, Shi W, Xue N, *et al.* Rationally designed anti-HIV peptides containing multifunctional domains as molecule probes for studying the mechanisms of action of the first and second generation HIV fusion inhibitors. J Biol Chem 2008; 283(44): 30376-84.

[77]   Labrosse B, Labernardiere JL, Dam E, *et al.* Baseline susceptibility of primary human immunodeficiency virus type 1 to entry inhibitors. J Virol 2003; 77(2): 1610-3.

[78]   Lalezari JP. Clinical safety and efficacy of enfuvirtide (T-20), a new fusion inhibitor. A review of the presentation at the satellite symposium "New hope: advancing care in HIV infection" at the 15th annual Association of Nurses in AIDS Care conference, November 2002. AIDS Read 2003; 13(3 Suppl): S9-13.

[79]   Jacobson JM, Lalezari JP, Thompson MA, *et al.* Phase 2a study of the CCR5 monoclonal antibody PRO 140 administered intravenously to HIV-infected adults. Antimicrob Agents Chemother 2010; 54(10): 4137-42.

[80]   Tenorio AR. The monoclonal CCR5 antibody PRO-140: the promise of once-weekly HIV therapy. Curr HIV/AIDS Rep 2011; 8(1): 1-3.

[81]   Pace CS, Fordyce MW, Franco D, Kao CY, Seaman MS, Ho DD. Anti-CD4 monoclonal antibody ibalizumab exhibits breadth and potency against HIV-1, with natural resistance mediated by the loss of a V5 glycan in envelope. J Acquir Immune Defic Syndr 2013; 62(1): 1-9.

[82]   Fletcher CV. Pharmacology of nucleoside reverse transcriptase inhibitors 2013 [updated 08 May 2013; cited 2014 21 June].

[83]   Rachlis AR. Zidovudine (Retrovir) update. CMAJ 1990; 143(11): 1177-85.

[84]   McLeod GX, Hammer SM. Zidovudine: five years later. Ann Intern Med 1992; 117(6): 487-501.

[85]   FDA. FDA notifications. NRTI Emtriva receives FDA approval. AIDS Alert 2003; 18(10): 131-2.

[86]   AIDSTreat. Abacavir (Ziagen) approval recommended 1998 [updated Nov 6No 306]. 4]. Available from: http: //www.ncbi.nlm.nih.gov/pubmed/11365961.

[87]   James JS. Lamivudine (3TC) approved for combination use with AZT. AIDS Treat News 1995(no 236): 1-5.

[88]   Piliero PJ. Pharmacokinetic properties of nucleoside/nucleotide reverse transcriptase inhibitors. J Acquir Immune Defic Syndr 2004; 37(Suppl 1): S2-S12.

[89]   Fung HB, Stone EA, Piacenti FJ. Tenofovir disoproxil fumarate: a nucleotide reverse transcriptase inhibitor for the treatment of HIV infection. Clin Ther 2002; 24(10): 1515-48.

[90]   Antoniou T, Park-Wyllie LY, Tseng AL. Tenofovir: a nucleotide analog for the management of human immunodeficiency virus infection. Pharmacotherapy 2003; 23(1): 29-43.

[91]   Grobler JA, Dornadula G, Rice MR, Simcoe AL, Hazuda DJ, Miller MD. HIV-1 reverse transcriptase plus-strand initiation exhibits preferential sensitivity to non-nucleoside reverse transcriptase inhibitors *in vitro*. J Biol Chem 2007; 282(11): 8005-10.

[92]   Graziani AL. Pharmacology of non-nucleoside reverse transcriptase inhibitors 2014 [updated Feb 07, 2014; cited 2014 June 23]. Available from: http: //www.uptodate.com/contents/pharmacology-of-non-nucleoside-reverse-transcriptase-inhibitors.

[93]   Beare KD, Coster MJ, Rutledge PJ. Diketoacid inhibitors of HIV-1 integrase: from L-708,906 to raltegravir and beyond. Curr Med Chem 2012; 19(8): 1177-92.

[94]   Bonnenfant S, Thomas CM, Vita C, *et al*. Styrylquinolines, integrase inhibitors acting prior to integration: a new mechanism of action for anti-integrase agents. J Virol 2004; 78(11): 5728-36.

[95]   Richman DD. HIV chemotherapy. Nature 2001; 410(6831): 995-1001.

[96]   Brower ET, Bacha UM, Kawasaki Y, Freire E. Inhibition of HIV-2 protease by HIV-1 protease inhibitors in clinical use. Chem Biol Drug Des 2008; 71(4): 298-305.

[97]   Yekkala R, Adams E, Van Schepdael A, Hoogmartens J. Quality control of protease inhibitors. J Pharm Sci 2008; 97(6): 2012-21.

[98]   Pokorna J, Machala L, Rezacova P, Konvalinka J. Current and Novel Inhibitors of HIV Protease. Viruses 2009; 1(3): 1209-39.

[99]   Dau B, Holodniy M. Novel targets for antiretroviral therapy: clinical progress to date. Drugs 2009.

[100]   He PA, Nie Z, Chen J, Chen J, Lv Z, Sheng Q, *et al*. Identification and characteristics of microRNAs from Bombyx mori. BMC genomics 2008; 9: 248.

[101]   Swaminathan S, Murray DD, and Kelleher A D. The role of microRNAs in HIV-1 pathogenesis and therapy. AIDS 2012; 26(11): 1325-34.

[102]   Wu L, Belasco JG. Examining the influence of microRNAs on translation efficiency and on mRNA deadenylation and decay. Methods in enzymology 2008; 449: 373-93.

[103]   Zhu H, Wu H, Liu X, *et al*. Role of MicroRNA miR-27a and miR-451 in the regulation of MDR1/P-glycoprotein expression in human cancer cells. Biochemical pharmacology 2008; 76(5): 582-8.

[104]   Brennecke J, Stark A, Russell RB, Cohen SM. Principles of MicroRNA–Target Recognition. PLoS Biology. 2005; 3(3).

[105]   Ahluwalia JK, Khan SZ, Soni K, *et al*. Human cellular microRNA hsa-miR-29a interferes with viral nef protein expression and HIV-1 replication. Retrovirology 2008; 5: 117.

[106]   Coleman SH, Day JR, Guatelli JC. The HIV-1 Nef protein as a target for antiretroviral therapy. Expert opinion on therapeutic targets 2001; 5(1): 1-22.

[107]   Huang J, Wang F, Argyris E, *et al*. Cellular microRNAs contribute to HIV-1 latency in resting primary CD4+ T lymphocytes. Nat Med 2007; 13: 1241.

[108]   Omoto S, Ito M, Tsutsumi Y, *et al*. HIV-1 nef suppression by virally encoded microRNA. Retrovirology 2004; 1: 44.

[109]   Pawlak EN, Dikeakos JD. HIV-1 Nef: a master manipulator of the membrane trafficking machinery mediating immune evasion. Biochimica et biophysica acta 2015; 1850(4): 733-41.

[110]   Sarkar R, Mitra D, Chakrabarti S. HIV-1 gp120 protein downregulates Nef induced IL-6 release in immature dentritic cells through interplay of DC-SIGN. PloS one 2013; 8(3): e59073.

[111]   Swaminathan G, Navas-Martin S, Martin-Garcia J. MicroRNAs and HIV-1 infection: antiviral activities and beyond. Journal of molecular biology 2014; 426(6): 1178-97.

[112]   Zhang Y, Fan M, Geng G, *et al*. A novel HIV-1-encoded microRNA enhances its viral replication by targeting the TATA box region. Retrovirology 2014; 11(1): 23.

[113]   Swaminathan G. Interplay between microRNAs, Toll-like receptors and HIV-1: Potential Implications in HIV-1 Replication and Chronic Immune Activation. Discovery Medicine 2014.

[114] Kim JH, Rerks-Ngarm S, Excler JL, Michael NL. HIV vaccines: lessons learned and the way forward. Current opinion in HIV and AIDS 2010; 5(5): 428-34.

[115] Wang LX. Bioorganic approaches towards HIV vaccine design. Current pharmaceutical design. 2003; 9(22): 1771-87.

[116] Wyatt R, Sodroski J. The HIV-1 envelope glycoproteins: fusogens, antigens, and immunogens. Science (New York, NY). 1998; 280(5371): 1884-8.

[117] Pinter A. Roles of HIV-1 Env variable regions in viral neutralization and vaccine development. Current HIV research 2007; 5(6): 542-53.

[118] Haynes BF, Montefiori DC. Aiming to induce broadly reactive neutralizing antibody responses with HIV-1 vaccine candidates. Expert review of vaccines 2006; 5(3): 347-63.

[119] KE. S, DH. B. A global approach to HIV-1 vaccine development. Immunol Rev 2013; 254(1): 295-304.

[120] Pantophlet R. Antibody epitope exposure and neutralization of HIV-1. Current pharmaceutical design. 2010; 16(33): 3729-43.

[121] Phogat S, Wyatt R. Rational modifications of HIV-1 envelope glycoproteins for immunogen design. Current pharmaceutical design 2007; 13(2): 213-27.

[122] Karlsson-Hedestam GB, Fouchier RA, Phogat S, Burton DR, Sodroski J, Wyatt RT. The challenges of eliciting neutralizing antibodies to HIV-1 and to influenza virus. Nature reviews Microbiology 2008; 6(2): 143-55.

[123] Haynes BF, Liao HX, Tomaras GD. Is developing an HIV-1 vaccine possible? Current opinion in HIV and AIDS. 2010; 5(5): 362-7.

[124] Hankins CA, Glasser JW, Chen RT. Modeling the impact of RV144-like vaccines on HIV transmission. Vaccine 2011; 29(36): 6069-71.

[125] de Souza MS, Ratto-Kim S, Chuenarom W, *et al.* The Thai phase III trial (RV144) vaccine regimen induces T cell responses that preferentially target epitopes within the V2 region of HIV-1 envelope. Journal of immunology (Baltimore, Md: 1950). 2012; 188(10): 5166-76.

[126] Guidelines for the Use of Antiretroviral Agents in HIV-1-Infected Adults and Adolescents [Internet]. 2014 [cited 20June2014]. Available from: http: //aidsinfo.nih.gov/guidelines/html/1/adult-and-adolescent-arv-guidelines/33/conclusion.

[127] HIV/AIDS: Summary of new recommendations [Internet]. 2013. Available from: http: //www.who.int/hiv/pub/guidelines/arv2013/intro/rag/en/index4.html.

[128] Ren J, Bird LE, Chamberlain PP, Stewart-Jones GB, Stuart DI, Stammers DK. Structure of HIV-2 reverse transcriptase at 2.35-A resolution and the mechanism of resistance to non-nucleoside inhibitors. Proceedings of the National Academy of Sciences of the United States of America. 2002; 99(22): 14410-5.

[129] Witvrouw M, Pannecouque C, Van Laethem K, Desmyter J, De Clercq E, Vandamme AM. Activity of non-nucleoside reverse transcriptase inhibitors against HIV-2 and SIV. Aids 1999; 13(12): 1477-83.

[130] Mallal S, Nolan D, Witt C, *et al.* Association between presence of HLA-B*5701, HLA-DR7, and HLA-DQ3 and hypersensitivity to HIV-1 reverse-transcriptase inhibitor abacavir. Lancet 2002; 359(9308): 727-32.

[131] Rodriguez-Novoa S, Soriano V. Current trends in screening across ethnicities for hypersensitivity to abacavir. Pharmacogenomics 2008; 9(10): 1531-41.

[132] Sanchez-Giron F, Villegas-Torres B, Jaramillo-Villafuerte K, *et al.* Association of the genetic marker for abacavir hypersensitivity HLA-B*5701 with HCP5 rs2395029 in Mexican Mestizos. Pharmacogenomics 2011; 12(6): 809-14.

[133] Offering information on HIV/AIDS Treatment, Prevention and Research [Internet]. 2013. Available from: http: //aidsinfo.nih.gov/education-materials/fact-sheets/19/73/the-hiv-life-cycle.

Appendix 1: Currently Registered Antiretroviral Agents

Generic Name	Year of FDA Approval
Nucleoside Reverse Transcriptase Inhibitors (NRTI)	
Emtricitabine (FTC)	2003
Enteric coated didanosine (ddI EC)	2000
Abacavir sulfate (ABC)	1998
Lamivudine (3TC)	1995
Stavudine (d4T)	1994
Zalcitabine dideoxycytidine (ddC) No longer marketed	1992
Didanosine (ddI)	1991
Zidovudine (AZT)	1987
Nucleotide Reverse Transcriptase Inhibitors (NtRTI)	
Tenofovir disoproxil fumarate (TDF)	2001
Non-nucleoside Reverse Transcriptase Inhibitors	
Rilpivirine	2011
Etravirine	2008
Efavirenz (EFV)	1998
Delavirdine (DLV)	1997
Nevirapine Immediate release (NVP)	1996
Nevirapine extended release	2011
Protease Inhibitors (PI	
Rilpivirine if VL<100,000	
Amprenavir (APV) (no longer marketed)	1999
Tipranavir (TPV)	2005
Indinavir (IDV)	1996
Saquinavir mesylate (SQV)	1995
Lopinavir + Ritonavir (LPV/RTV)	2000
Fosamprenavir Calcium(FOS-APV)	2003
Ritonavir (RTV)	1996
Darunavir	2006
Atazanavir sulphate (ATV)	2003
Atazanavir + Ritonavir	
Nelfinavir mesylate (NFV)	1997
HIV Entry Inhibitors	
Enfuvirtide (T-20)	2003
Maraviroc	2007
Integrase Inhibitors	
Raltegravir	2007
Elvitegravir	
Dolutegravir	2013
Others	
Cobicistat (Booster)	

CHAPTER 2

HIV-1 Entry Inhibitors

Joshua R. Sawyer[1,2,3], Charles S. Venuto[1,4] and Gene D. Morse[1,2,4,*]

[1]*Translational Pharmacology Research Core, New York State Center of Excellence in Bioinformatics and Life Sciences, USA;* [2]*School of Pharmacy and Pharmaceutical Sciences, University at Buffalo, NY, USA;* [3]*Erie County Medical Center Corporation, Buffalo NY USA;* [4]*Center for Human Experimental Therapeutics, University of Rochester, Rochester NY, USA*

Abstract: Current therapeutic intervention in HIV infection relies upon over 30 different therapeutic options. Despite the efficacy shown by these drugs, clinicians are confronted with an unexpected frequency of adverse effects and resistance, including transmitted resistance. There is now a great need for new drugs with reduced toxicity, increased activity against drug-resistant viruses and a greater capacity to reach tissue sanctuaries of the virus. Drugs that target the interactions between the HIV envelope and the cellular receptor complex are a 'new entry' into the scenario of HIV therapy and have recently raised great interest because of their activity against multidrug-resistant viruses. Two such drugs include maraviroc, a CCR5 antagonist, and enfuvirtide, a fusion inhibitor, both of which work *via* separate mechanisms to block the entry of HIV into the cell. The clinical pharmacology, and studies of efficacy and safety of these two agents, and investigational drugs within this class, are described in this current chapter.

Keywords: Entry inhibitors, Maraviroc, Enfuvirtide, Fusion, CCR5-antagonism, Albuvirtide, T-20, Cenicriviroc, HIV pharmacology, Antiretroviral therapy, ART.

INTRODUCTION

Currently, 35 antiretroviral medications, or combination antiretroviral tablets are approved by the United States Food and Drug Administration (FDA) for the treatment of HIV/AIDS. With the advent of highly active antiretroviral therapy (HAART), patients in the United States who were living with HIV/AIDS saw a decline in morbidity and mortality for the first time since cases of rare cancer and pneumonia were seen in gay men in 1981 [1, 2]. However, further concern soon arose regarding a need for strict adherence to these complex medication regimens in the face of serious adverse drug reactions [3], and the emergence of drug resistance [4]. An increase in the transmission of drug-resistant virus also became

*Corresponding author Gene D. Morse:** Translational Pharmacology Research Core, NYS Center of Excellence in Bioinformatics and Life Sciences, 701 Ellicott Street, Buffalo, NY 14203, USA; Tel: 716-881-7464; Fax: 716-849-6890; E-mail: emorse@buffalo.edu

apparent [5]. Even mild and transient adverse events can negatively impact on a patient's quality of life [6]. A need for effective medications that had minimal adverse events and had different mechanisms of action, and thus resistance profiles became apparent. An expanded understanding of the viral life cycle of the human immunodeficiency virus (HIV) has allowed for an increased number of antiretroviral medications available in the armamentarium in the fight against HIV/AIDS.

Before the virus even enters the cell, a complex interplay between viral envelop and host cell membrane must transpire [7, 8]. Infection cannot occur without the HIV surface envelope glycoprotein (gp120) attaching to a CD4 receptor that is found on T-lymphocytes, macrophages, dendritic cells and other cells involved in the human immune response. This interaction induces a conformational change, revealing a chemokine co-receptor binding site on gp120. Chemokines are small (8 – 10 kilodaltons) proteins critical to mediating immune cell migration. They exert their biological effect by binding to chemokine receptors, which are G protein-coupled receptors found on the surface of different immune cells. Although nearly 20 different chemokine receptors have been identified in humans, only two have been found to be relevant to the pathogenesis of HIV-1 infection; these are CXCR4 and CCR5 of the host cell [9]. After binding to both the CD4 receptor and the co-receptor, a further conformational change allows the viral envelope to come into direct contact with the host cell's membrane. A fusion peptide found on the viral particle known as glycoprotein (gp41), pierces the host cell. Repeat sequences in gp41, known as heptad repeats 1 and 2 (HR1 and HR2) consist of the amino acids leucine or isoleucine at every seventh position over six helical turns [10]. These "leucine zippers" interact with each other, leading to the collapse of the extracellular portion of gp41, and fusion of the viral envelope and the host cell membrane. The protein-containing core of the virus enters the host cell's cytoplasm, and infection commences (Fig. **1**).

Understanding the mechanisms of viral entry into the host cell has led to new paths of investigation seeking to create antiretroviral agents with novel mechanisms of action, which block this crucial step in the infectious process. Ongoing research probes each of the various aspects of entry described above. Currently, two antiretroviral agents, each with a unique mechanism of action have been approved, which inhibit the entry of HIV into the host cell.

Host Cell and HIV ⟶ CD4 Binding ⟶ Co-receptor binding

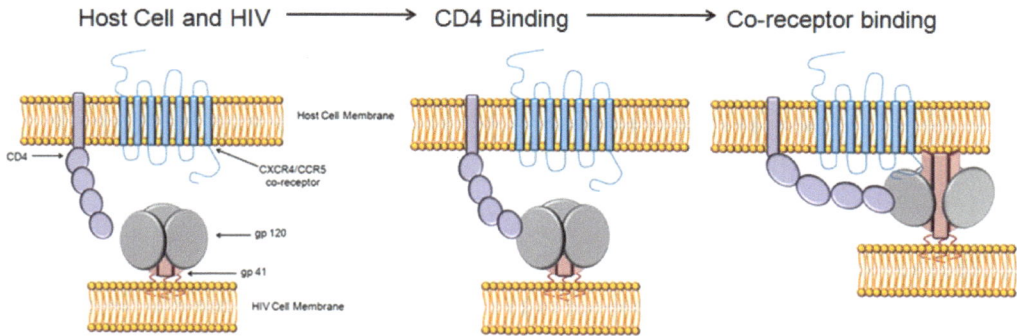

Fig. (1). Entry of HIV into the host cell is initiated by attachment between the CD4 receptor on the host cell and gp-120 of the virus. Next, co-receptor binding occurs between chemokine co-receptors, CXCR4/CCR5 of the host cell, and gp-120, which undergoes conformational changes. These changes allow gp-41 to attach to host cell membrane and mediate fusion (not depicted) between the two membranes for HIV cell entry. [Adapted from Wilen *et al*. Cold Spring Harb Perspect Med 2012].

ENFUVIRTIDE (T-20)

Mechanism of Action

Enfuvirtide was the first entry inhibitor approved by the FDA on March 13, 2003. It is indicated in combination with other antiretroviral agents in the treatment of experienced patients with evidence of HIV replication despite ongoing antiretroviral therapy [11]. It is a 36 amino acid poly-peptide that is produced synthetically as an analogue to an aspect of HR2 of gp41 [12]. The agent binds to HR1, preventing the interaction between HR1 and HR2, thus preventing the conformational change that allows fusion of the viral cell envelope to that of the host cell membrane. Unlike chemokine co-receptor antagonists, which will be discussed below, enfuvirtide appears to be active against viruses that utilize the CCR5 co-receptor (R5 tropic viruses), the CXCR4 co-receptor (X4 tropic viruses), or both co-receptors (dual/mixed, or D/M tropic viruses) [13].

Pharmacokinetics

Absorption and Distribution in Adults

Enfuvirtide is administered as a subcutaneous injection, and following a single dose of 90 mg SQ, the agent has a small volume of distribution of 5.48L [14]. It is highly protein bound (92%) to albumin and α-1 acid glycoprotein, and exposure appears to be linearly dose dependent [15]. The agent has a bioavailability of 84.3% [14]. The bioavailability does differ slightly depending upon the site of administration, but this has not been noted to be clinically significant, and SQ injection into the arm, thigh or abdomen is appropriate [15].

Metabolism and Elimination in Adults

As a peptide, enfuvirtide undergoes protein catabolism. It undergoes hydrolysis at the C-terminal phenylalanine residue, which results in a minimally active deaminated metabolite [15], and it is believed that this metabolite undergoes further catabolism to be eliminated. The mean half-life of this agent is 3.8 hours [15, 16].

Effect of Sex, Body Weight, Age and Race on Pharmacokinetics

Post hoc analysis of pharmacokinetic data from TORO-1 and TORO-2 phase III trials (described below) describes a 20% lower clearance in female patients utilizing enfuvirtide compared to males [15]. Clearance also increases with the increase in body weight [15]. Race does not appear to influence the rate of clearance of enfuvirtide. These differences in clearance do not appear to be clinically significant and dose adjustments are not recommended.

Pharmacokinetics in Pediatric Patients

When administered a dose of 2 mg/kg twice daily, enfuvirtide pharmacokinetics appear to be similar to those seen in adults given a dose of 90 mg twice daily [15, 16].

Pharmacokinetics in Pregnant Women

There is an inadequate data on the pharmacokinetics of enfuvirtide in pregnant women.

Dosing and Administration

Enfuvirtide is given as a 90 mg (1 ml) subcutaneous injection twice daily. Because enfuvirtide is a synthetic peptide, oral administration is not possible, due to catabolism by gastrointestinal peptidases. Injection sites should be rotated between upper arms, thighs and abdomen, and should not be given in an area where an injection site reaction from previous injections is evident.

A study comparing 180 mg of enfuvirtide given as two subcutaneous injections once daily to 90 mg of enfuvirtide given subcutaneously twice daily, demonstrated a 49% higher maximum observed plasma concentration within a dosing interval and a 57% lower pre-dose plasma concentration for once daily injections [17]. The authors concluded that there was a trend toward less virologic efficacy with the once daily dosing of enfuvirtide *versus* twice daily injections. Given the small sample size, additional studies are required before once daily dosing can be considered in patients utilizing this agent.

Enfuvirtide does not appear to require dose adjustments in patients with renal dysfunction, and the drug is only minimally cleared by intermittent hemodialysis [18]. Although pharmacokinetic analysis has not occurred in patients with hepatic dysfunction, the medication is not cleared *via* hepatic enzymes and does not appear to need dose adjustment based upon the changes in hepatic function [19].

Enfuvirtide is a pregnancy category B drug. Data regarding this agent's use in pregnancy is limited [20-22] and further research is needed to ensure safe and effective use in pregnant women. It is unknown if enfuvirtide is excreted in breast milk. However, because of the unknown potential for adverse events, and the risk of transmission of HIV through breast milk, women should refrain from breast feeding their child while on enfuvirtide.

Adverse Events

The most common adverse event in patients taking enfuvirtide has been injection site reactions (ISRs). These events are experienced by 98% of patients using enfuvirtide, and include pain and discomfort (96%), erythema (91%), nodules or cysts (80%), pruritus (65%), and ecchymosis (52%). These events typically occurred in the first week of enfuvirtide use and there is no evidence to suggest that ISRs are more frequent over time [23-25]. In clinical trials [24, 25], only a small number discontinued treatment with enfuvirtide due to adverse ISRs. Needle free systems and other mechanisms have been studied as effective means of delivering enfuvirtide with less injection reactions [26, 27], however feasibility of their use are in question due to cost and availability of these products.

In addition to ISR, combined TORO trial data suggest 75% of patients in the control arm experienced a treatment related adverse event compared with 78% of patients treated with enfuvirtide [24, 25]. The only adverse events experienced at a rate of more than 5% in the enfuvirtide treatment group were peripheral neuropathy and decreased appetite.

Hypersensitivity reactions may occur with enfuvirtide, and these reactions may reappear upon further challenge with the medication. Symptoms of the hypersensitivity reaction include fever, chills, rash, nausea, vomiting, hypotension or elevated serum liver enzymes, or any combination of these symptoms.

In the event when a provider considers the utilization of enfuvirtide in combination with other antiretroviral agents in a heavily treatment experienced patient with HIV, quality of life and adherence to this medication is improved with continuous support and education [28].

Monitoring

Enfuvirtide does not appear to be associated with mitochondrial toxicities or abnormalities in blood lipid or glucose levels [29]. Clinical trials suggest monitoring for neutropenia, anemia, and elevated liver transaminases [24, 25]. As with all antiretroviral agents, efficacy of the drug requires monitoring of CD4 count and HIV plasma RNA levels.

Drug Interactions

Enfuvirtide does not appear to inhibit or induce CYP450 isoenzymes [30]. Clinically significant drug interactions were not observed when enfuvirtide was given concomitantly with rifampin or ritonavir [31]. Simultaneous use of enfuvirtide with tipranavir/ritonavir resulted in notably higher tipranavir and ritonavir trough concentrations than in patients taking tipranavir/ritonavir without enfuvirtide [32]. The mechanism of this interaction is not known, and manufacturers do not recommend decreasing the dose of the protease inhibitors when used with enfuvirtide.

Clinical Pharmacology

Two phase-III, randomized, open-label trials were conducted to determine the efficacy and safety of enfuvirtide (T-20) in the treatment of HIV/AIDS [24, 25]. The T-20 *vs.* Optimized Regimen Only Study 1 (TORO1) [24] was conducted in sites in the United States, Canada and Brazil, and included treatment experienced patients with at least six months of previous treatment with three classes of antiretroviral therapy (nucleoside reverse transcriptase inhibitors, non-nucleoside reverse transcriptase inhibitors, and protease inhibitors), resistance to drugs in these classes, or both. The patients had to have an HIV viral load of at least 5000 copies/ml. A total of 501 patients were randomized to receive enfuvirtide plus optimized background regimen *versus* optimized background regimen alone. At baseline, both arms were similar in demographics, previous antiretroviral therapy, HIV viral load and CD4 count. At twenty-four weeks, the enfuvirtide group had a decrease in plasma viral load of 1.696 log10 copies/ml, while the control arm had a decrease in viral load of 0.764 log10 copies/ml (p<0.001). The mean CD4 cell increase was 76 cells/mm^3 in the enfuvirtide arm *versus* 32 cells/mm^3 in the control arm (p<0.001). The drug appeared safe, with limited treatment related to systemic adverse events. As stated previously, 98.2% of patients did report injection site reactions. Decreased appetite and peripheral neuropathy were the only other adverse events that occurred in at least five percent of patients on enfuvirtide.

A study of similar design (TORO2) [25] was completed with patients from sites throughout Europe and Australia. Baseline characteristics were well matched. At twenty-four weeks, the enfuvirtide arm had a decrease in plasma viral load of 1.429 log10 copies/ml *versus* a decline of 0.648 log10 copies/ml in the control arm (p<0.001). The average CD4 increase was 65.5 cells/mm^3 in the study arm *versus* only 38 cells/mm^3 in the control arm (p=0.02). Nearly 98% of patients in the enfuvirtide arm experienced localized injection site reactions. While the enfuvirtide arm experienced adverse reactions more often than the control arm, no adverse reaction other than injection site reactions occurred in more than five percent of patients on the study drug.

When safety analysis of the combined study populations was done, bacterial pneumonias were also more likely in the enfuvirtide arm, and the difference was significant (p=0.02).Causality could not be proven. Sepsis also appeared more likely in patients taking enfuvirtide, though this was not statistically significant. Two cases of hypersensitivity reaction occurred in TORO1 [24], and both occurred again upon re-challenge to enfuvirtide. The most frequent adverse events leading to withdrawal in both studies were nausea, vomiting or diarrhea, though these adverse events occurred in both treatment arms, and were not statistically significant in either arm.

Resistance

Resistance to enfuvirtide occurs rapidly in the face of virologic failure, and continuing enfuvirtide in a patient failing therapy leads to the selection of additional resistance mutations [32]. In phase III trials, amino acid substitutions in HR1 on gp41 were associated with decreased phenotypic susceptibility to enfuvirtide [33]. Mutations that have been noted to cause resistance to enfuvirtide include: G36D/S, I37V, V38A/M/E, Q39R, Q40H, N42T, and N43D [34]. An enfuvirtide resistance associated mutation on HR2, S138A, has also been seen in patients failing enfuvirtide [35].

Genotypic assays are available commercially that test the gp41 for mutations that may decrease susceptibility to enfuvirtide.

FUSION INHIBITORS IN DEVELOPMENT

Albuvirtide is a fusion inhibitor that binds to the HIV gp41 with a half-life of eleven days [36]. In early monotherapy studies in treatment naïve patients, doses of 160 mg or 320 mg were given *via* intravenous injection on days 1, 2, and 3 and then were given weekly on days 8 and 15. The average decline in plasma RNA levels were 0.68 log10 with the 160 mg dose and 1.05 log10 with the 320 mg dose. The drug appeared to suppress HIV viral load for more than six days, but viral rebound was noted in all cases after day fifteen. Albuvirtide appears active against enfuvirtide resistant strains of HIV [37].

CHEMOKINE CO-RECEPTOR ANTAGONISTS

Utilizing a second step in the process of viral entry into the host cell, chemokine co-receptor antagonists block the binding of the virus to CCR5 or CXCR4 co-receptor sites. After initial binding of gp120 to the CD4 receptors, a conformational change occurs that exposes a co-receptor protein. Amino acid sequences V1-V2 and V3 in the HIV envelope protein gp120 establish the use of CCR5 or CXCR4 co-receptors, and the expression of either CCR5 or CXCR4 on host cells determines their vulnerability to infection by the virus [8]. In addition, dual/mixed (DM) tropic viruses are able to utilize both CCR5 and CXCR4 co-receptors, and a single patient may harbor a combination of CCR5 and CXCR4 tropic virus strains. Viruses that are R5 tropic are the most common during acute phase of HIV infection and are seen in a majority of treatment naïve patients [38]. Viruses that are X4 tropic arise in later stages of infection upon treatment experience, and involve faster replication rate, and thus disease progression [39].

Tropism Testing

Standard tropism testing involves phenotypic assays, which utilize the HIV-1 envelope gene sequences from a patient's virus inserted into a laboratory virus modified to contain a reporter gene that detects infectivity of the recombinant viral product [40]. The reassembled virus then is used to infect laboratory derived cells that consist of CD4 receptors and CCR5 or CXCR4 receptors. In the presence of a co-receptor antagonist, the virus infects cells that utilize the co-receptor that has not been blocked. The Trophile assay (Monogram Biosciences) reports results as R5, X4, or dual/mixed (D/M), and assists the clinician by reporting whether utilization of a CCR5 antagonist is expected to be efficacious. The original Trophile assay was able to detect X4 viruses in patients provided that at least ten percent of the circulating HIV strains were X4 tropic. A later generation Trophile assay with increased sensitivity for X4 was created which is better able to detect patients who are D/M tropic. This Trophile assay with enhanced sensitivity has since replaced the first generation Trophile assay and is able to detect X4 variants if they comprise at least 0.3% of the total virus population [40, 41]. A genotypic assay is available and is the currently recommended method to determine viral tropism in Europe [42].

Review of the available literature on the efficacy and safety of CCR5 antagonists must be undertaken with caution regarding the revised clinical use of phenotypic tropism testing, as population reanalysis of patients who were originally deemed as having R5 tropic viruses and placed on a CCR5 antagonist showed that many of those who failed the CCR5 antagonist were actually D/M tropic using the enhanced sensitivity Trophile assay [43].

CCR5 Antagonists

Despite halting clinical trials involving aplaviroc, one of the initial CCR5 antagonists in development, due to reports of severe liver toxicity [44], several other agents in this class are under investigation. Maraviroc has been approved by the US FDA for use in combination with other antiretrovirals in the treatment of HIV/AIDS in both treatment experienced and treatment naïve patients.

MARAVIROC (UK-427857)

Mechanism of Action

In patients with CCR5 tropic strains, maraviroc is a selective and noncompetitive antagonist of the chemokine CCR5 receptor. Upon interaction with the CCR5 receptor, maraviroc inhibits the viral envelope peptide – co-receptor binding that is necessary to allow viral fusion and entry into host cells. The medication has limited effect in patients who harbor CXCR4 tropic viruses or D/M tropic viruses.

Pharmacokinetics

Maraviroc is a substrate for both CYP450 3A isoenzymes and P-glycoprotein efflux transport systems.

Absorption and Distribution in Adults

Maraviroc is administered as an oral tablet, and bioavailability of a single 300 mg dose is predicted to be 33% based upon the bioavailability of a single 100 mg dose being 23%. An increase in peak concentrations and absolute bioavailability is not proportionate to dose given [45]. Mean maximum concentrations occur between 0.5 to 4 hours after single doses across the dosing range. Administering a single maraviroc 300 mg dose with a high fat meal reduces the peak concentration and bioavailability of the drug by 33%, and appears to reduce the peak concentration and bioavailability of maraviroc by 60% and 40% respectively when this agent is given as 150 mg orally twice daily [46]. There does not appear to be an effect on the antiviral activity of maraviroc when administered with high fat meals, and as such, the medication can be taken with or without food.

Maraviroc is moderately bound (76%) to albumin and α-1-acid glycoprotein, and has a volume of distribution of 194L. The medication appears to concentrate in vaginal secretions and tissue at higher levels than in plasma [47], and has been reported to also rapidly distribute into seminal fluids, rectal tissue and the central nervous system [48, 49].

Metabolism and Excretion in Adults

Maraviroc is metabolized by the CYP450 3A isoenzymes into metabolites without antiretroviral activity. The major metabolite is a secondary amine formed from N-dealkylation, but other metabolites are formed as a result of mono-oxidation [46]. Eight percent of maraviroc is excreted unchanged in urine, 25% is excreted unchanged in feces and the inactive metabolites serve as the remainder of excreted drug. In healthy volunteers the drug has a half-life of 14 to 18 hours.

Effect of Sex, Body Weight, Age and Race on Pharmacokinetics

Sex at birth, body weight, and race do not appear to alter pharmacokinetics, though formal pharmacokinetic studies have not occurred. In clinical trials, there were an insufficient number of patients younger than 16 years of age or greater than 65 years of age to determine the pharmacokinetic differences in these populations [46].

Pharmacokinetics in Pediatric Patients

The pharmacokinetics of maraviroc has not been established in patients less than sixteen years of age.

Pharmacokinetics in Pregnant Women

There are no pharmacokinetic studies of maraviroc in human pregnancy [50].

Dosing and Administration

In the United States, maraviroc is approved for use in combination with other antiretroviral agents in the treatment of HIV/AIDS in both treatment naïve and treatment experienced patients. It is not indicated for the treatment of patients with CXCR4 or D/M tropic strains of HIV. In adults, the dosage of maraviroc is 150 mg, 300mg, or 600mg twice daily, dependent upon drug interactions between maraviroc and coadministered medications (Table 1). The medication can be taken in fed or fasting states without clinical significance upon antiviral efficacy or safety of the drug.

In an effort to find a safe and efficacious regimen that does not contain nucleoside reverse transcriptase inhibitors (NRTIs), which are known to have several adverse events related to long term use [51, 52], research is ongoing involving the use of a boosted protease inhibitor with once daily maraviroc as a viable option. Two such options are ritonavir boosted atazanavir plus once daily maraviroc [53], and ritonavir boosted darunavir plus once daily maraviroc [54].

In a randomized open label study comparing atazanavir (300 mg with 100 mg of ritonavir) plus tenofovir/emtricitabine (300mg/200mg) or maraviroc (150 mg) daily [53], 82% of the tenofovir/emtricitabine control arm had viral loads under 50 copies/ml compared with 67.8% of the patients in the maraviroc treatment arm at ninety-six weeks of therapy. Gains in CD4 cells were similar in patients treated with tenofovir/emtricitabine (+264 cells/ml) *versus* those treated with maraviroc (+240 cells/ml). Serious adverse events were reported in 18% of patients in the tenofovir/emtricitabine arm and in 21.7% of those in the maraviroc arm. Creatinine clearance decreased more in the tenofovir/emtricitabine arm (-18 ml/min) than in the maraviroc group (-5.5 ml/min). Hyperbilirubinemia was less likely in the tenofovir/emtricitabine arm, a fact that study investigators attributed to lower atazanavir concentrations with tenofovir.

In a multi-center, single-arm open label pilot study twenty-four treatment naïve patients were treated with darunavir (800 mg) boosted with ritonavir (100 mg) plus maraviroc (150mg) once daily [54]. At twenty-four weeks four patients had virological failure, and three of these patients had pretreatment viral loads greater than 100,000 copies/ml.

A post hoc analysis of the MOTIVATE trials (described below) compared the efficacy of maraviroc given 150 mg once or 150 mg twice daily with boosted protease inhibitors (other than fosamprenavir or tipranavir) at week 48 [55]. Similar proportions of patients in the once daily maraviroc arm (45.5%) and patients in the twice daily maraviroc arm (47.4%) had viral loads less than 50 copies/ml when compared with placebo (16.5%). The investigators concluded that once daily maraviroc as part of a treatment regimen containing boosted protease inhibitors may offer treatment experienced patients treatment regimens at decreased costs. Further data is required before such dosing strategies can be recommended.

Maraviroc is metabolized through the liver, and while the efficacy and safety of maraviroc in HIV positive patients with hepatic impairment have not been studied, a clinician should be vigilant if prescribing the medication in a patient with hepatic impairment. An open label, non-randomized single-center parallel group study of HIV negative patients with mild, moderate, and normal hepatic dysfunction, (n=24) was conducted in which all patients received a single dose of maraviroc 300 mg [56]. Despite minor changes in pharmacokinetic parameters in patients with hepatic dysfunction, the investigators concluded that current data did not support the requirement for a dose adjustment in this patient population.

A single 300 mg dose maraviroc study compared the pharmacokinetics of maraviroc in HIV negative patients with severe renal impairment or end-stage renal disease to HIV negative patients with normal renal function. When adjusting for dosage, peak concentrations and bioavailability was higher in patients with severe renal impairment or end-stage renal disease. The manufacturer does not recommend dose adjustments in renal disease for patients who are not on inducers or inhibitors of CYP450 3A, unless the patient complains of symptomatic postural hypotension [46]. In these patients, suggested dosing is 300 mg twice daily if creatinine clearance is greater than or equal to 30 ml/min. If used in combination with a strong CYP450 3A inhibitor, and the creatinine clearance is greater than or equal to 30 ml/min, the dose of maraviroc is recommended to be 150 mg twice daily (Table **1**). If the creatinine clearance is less than 30 ml/min, use of maraviroc is not recommended. If used in combination with strong CYP450 3A inducers and the creatinine clearance is greater than or equal to 30 ml/min, the suggested dose of maraviroc is 600 mg twice daily. The drug does not appear to be cleared by intermittent hemodialysis.

Table 1. Recommended dosing of Maraviroc with CYP450 3A modulators.

CYP450 3A Modulators	Creatinine Clearance =/>30 ml/min
None	Maraviroc 300 mg twice daily
Strong CYP3A Inducers	Maraviroc 600 mg twice daily
Strong CYP3A Inhibitors	Maraviroc 150 mg twice daily

Adverse Events

Maraviroc appears to be well tolerated. Upper respiratory tract infections (55% in maraviroc arms *versus* 40% in control arms), with cough (14%) or fever (13%), rash (11%) and dizziness were the most likely adverse events noted by treatment experienced patients in clinical trials. Though causality could not be established between the use of maraviroc and these events, they did appear to occur more frequently with maraviroc 300 mg twice daily than in patients in the control arm. There was a longer duration of treatment exposure in patients in the maraviroc arms, and when this was taken into account, the exposure-adjusted frequency of these events was 133 per 100 subject years in both maraviroc and control arms.

There were no significant differences in the incidence of severe hepatotoxicity between maraviroc and control arms in studies with maraviroc. Less than 2% of patients presented with hepatic cirrhosis, hepatic failure, portal vein thrombosis, jaundice or elevated serum transaminase levels. In these studies, there was also no evidence of drug induced hepatotoxicity in patients who were co-infected with hepatitis B or hepatitis C. In post approval surveillance, hepatitis has been reported in some patients receiving maraviroc, and prior to the development of overt hepatitis, drug reaction with eosinophilia and systemic symptoms (DRESS) had been seen. Because of this, a blackbox warning has been included in the prescribing information of maraviroc [46].

In clinical trials, 11 patients (1.3%) who received maraviroc experienced a cardiovascular event including myocardial infarction, and no events were reported in patients in the control arms. The patients who experienced a cardiac event generally had known cardiac risk factors or disease prior to maraviroc use, and causality cannot be assessed.

Monitoring

Maraviroc does not require special monitoring. A sub analysis of studies done in treatment naïve patients using zidovudine/lamivudine (300mg/150mg) twice daily plus efavirenz 600 mg daily or maraviroc 300 mg daily, suggests that maraviroc does not elevate serum triglycerides, low density lipoprotein (LDL) or total cholesterol [57]. As with all antiretroviral agents, efficacy of maraviroc can be monitored by periodic evaluation of CD4 count and plasma HIV viral load.

Drug Interactions

Maraviroc is not an inhibitor or an inducer of CYP450 enzymes and thus is not expected to alter serum levels of simultaneously coadministered medications that are metabolized by these enzymes [58].

Maraviroc is a substrate of CYP 450 3A and P-glycoprotein, and systemic exposure of this agent is affected by coadministered medications which are inhibitors or inducers of the CYP 450 3A isoenzymes or the P-glycoprotein efflux transporter. Protease inhibitors combined with low dose ritonavir (with the exception of tipranavir) are inhibitors of CYP 3A, and concentrations of maraviroc are increased. As such, in the presence of a strong CYP 3A inhibitor, maraviroc dosing is decreased to 150 mg twice daily (Table 1). Efavirenz and etravirine are inducers of CYP 3A, and concentrations are decreased by these drugs. In the presence of a strong CYP 3A inducer, maraviroc dosing is increased to 600 mg twice daily. Rifampicin is an inducer of CYP 3A and decreases the peak concentrations and bioavailability of maraviroc [59], and guidelines suggest increasing the dose of maraviroc to 600 mg twice daily. Ketoconazole is a potent inhibitor of CYP 3A, and guidelines recommend decreasing coadministered maraviroc to 150 mg twice daily [60].

There do not appear to be clinically significant drug interactions between maraviroc and sulfamethoxazole/trimethoprim, tenofovir, raltegravir, zidovudine, lamivudine, midazolam or oral contraceptives levonorgestrel or ethinyl estradiol in HIV negative adults [61-63].

Clinical Pharmacology

Treatment Experienced Patients

Two double blind, placebo-controlled, phase III trials known as Maraviroc *versus* Optimized Therapy in Viremic Antiretroviral Treatment-Experienced Patients (MOTIVATE) 1 and MOTIVATE 2, were conducted in patients who had R5 tropic HIV [64]. Patients had resistance to three antiretroviral drug classes and had HIV viral loads greater than 5000 copies/ml. One thousand forty-nine patients were randomized to receive optimized background therapy (OBT) alone, or OBT in combination with once daily maraviroc or twice daily maraviroc. At 48 weeks, change in HIV viral load from baseline was greater with once daily maraviroc and twice daily maraviroc when compared to placebo (decreases of -1.66, - 1.82 and - 0.8 log10, respectively in MOTIVATE 1 and -1.72, - 1.87, and -0.76 log10, respectively in MOTIVATE 2). Patients with undetectable viral loads less than 50 copies/ml were more likely in the maraviroc once and twice daily arms *versus* placebo as well (42% and 47% *versus* 16% in MOTIVATE 1 and 45% and 45% *versus* 18% in MOTIVATE 2, p<0.001). Increases in CD4 count were also greater in patients randomized to receive once or twice daily maraviroc *versus* placebo in both studies (increases of 113 and 122 *versus* 54 in MOTIVATE 1 and increases of 122 and 128 *versus* 69 in MOTIVATE 2, p<0.001). Combined analysis of the 96 week data revealed continued viral loads of less than 50 copies/ml in patients on once daily maraviroc and twice daily maraviroc (39% and 41%) [65]. At 96 weeks, the most common adverse events in patients on maraviroc were nasopharyngitis, upper respiratory infections, rash and dizziness. Analysis of the incidence of malignancies at week 48 and presented at 96 weeks did not reveal a difference between maraviroc or placebo arms of the studies.

Treatment Naïve Patients

The Maraviroc *versus* Efavirenz in Treatment Naïve Patients (MERIT) study compared maraviroc with efavirenz, both in the presence of backbone nucleoside reverse transcriptase inhibitors zidovudine/lamivudine [66]. Patients enrolled in this study had R5 tropic viruses. Patients were randomized to receive efavirenz 600 mg, once daily maraviroc 300 mg daily, or maraviroc 300 mg twice daily; however the maraviroc once daily arm was halted early for not meeting pre-specified non-inferiority criteria. Nine hundred and seventeen patients were randomized to receive study drug, and 174 were enrolled in the maraviroc once daily arm, and thus were not analyzed. Seven hundred and twenty one patients were treated, and at 48 weeks, maraviroc was noninferior for <400 copies/ml (70.6% for maraviroc *versus* 73.1% for efavirenz), but not for <50 copies/ml (65.3% *versus* 69.3%). Interestingly more maraviroc patients discontinued treatment due to lack of efficacy (11.9% *versus* 4.2%) but more patients discontinued efavirenz due to adverse events (4.2% *versus* 13.6%). The interim analysis was repeated post hoc to discern the likely role of enhanced sensitivity tropism testing, and 107 (15%) of the 721 patients treated had a D/M virus using the more sensitive screening assay. Of the 614 patients with confirmed R5 virus, reanalysis reduced the rate of discontinuation of maraviroc for lack of efficacy from 11.9% to 9.3%. Patients on maraviroc had greater increases in CD4 count from baseline (+170 cells/ml) than those on efavirenz (+144 cell/ml, p = 0.08).

Bronchitis and nasopharyngitis were more common in patients taking maraviroc than in those taking efavirenz, but diarrhea, nausea, dizziness, abnormal dreams and rash were more common on efavirenz. After 96 weeks of treatment, investigators evaluated the durability of virologic response and analyzed safety of maraviroc [67]. A total of 58.8% of patients on maraviroc twice daily reached viral loads < 50 copies/ml compared to 62.7% of patients on efavirenz, and there was a similar proportion of time to loss of virologic response respondents who obtained viral loads < 50 copies/ml (60.5% *versus* 60.7%, with maraviroc and efavirenz, respectively). Mean increases in CD4 count were again greater in those patients taking maraviroc (+212cell/ml) than in those taking efavirenz (+171 cells/ml, p=0.01). At both weeks 48 and 96, there were fewer treatment-related adverse events in the maraviroc arm, most of which occurred within the first 48 weeks, and no new findings were revealed between weeks 48 and 96.

Further reanalysis of both MOTIVATE data and MERIT data using deep V3 gene sequencing for HIV-1 tropism [68, 69], suggesting that, had this approach been utilized as the original screening method, greater numbers of patients would have been found to have been D/M tropic, and hence excluded from the studies.

Pre-exposure Prophylaxis Treatment

Orally administered maraviroc is undergoing clinical safety and tolerability testing in HIV-uninfected at-risk individuals with or without tenofovir and/or emtricitabine as a potential agent for pre-exposure prophylaxis treatment [70]. In order for entry inhibitors to prove effective in preventing transmission, drug concentrations must reach potent levels at the cell membrane of immune targets in the genital and/or rectal tracts. Several pharmacokinetic studies in healthy volunteers have demonstrated maraviroc levels within the cervicovaginal fluid and seminal plasma to exceed the protein free 90% inhibitory concentration (0.5 ng/mL) of maraviroc [71, 72]. Exposure of unbound maraviroc in the cervicovaginal fluid, rectal tissue, and seminal plasma were as high as 2.7-fold, 26-fold, and 2-fold, greater than blood plasma exposure, respectively.

Resistance

Failure of a maraviroc containing regimen may be the result of selection of CXCR4 tropic virus, but documented resistance to maraviroc has been noted, even in patients who maintain a CCR5 tropic viral strain. Mutations in the V3 loop of envelope gp120 may lead to reduced susceptibility to maraviroc [73, 74]. Mutations in non-V3 regions of gp120 have also been investigated regarding their potential to cause resistance to maraviroc [75].

CCR5 and CXCR4 ANTAGONIST IN DEVELOPMENT

There are several CCR5 and CXCR4 antagonists under investigation (Table **2**).

Table 2. CCR5 and CXCR4 antagonists currently in mid-stage development.

Drug Name (Company)	Mechanism of Action	Latest Clinical Phase of Development
AMD070 (Genzyme Corp.)	CXCR4 antagonist	II
INCB-9471 (Incyte Corp.)	CCR5 antagonist	II
Cenicriviroc (Takeda; Tobira Therapeutics)	CCR5 antagonist	II
PRO-140 (CytoDyn Inc.)	CCR5 antagonist	II

CONFLICT OF INTEREST

The authors confirm that this chapter contents have no conflict of interest.

ACKNOWLEDGEMENTS

Declared none.

REFERENCES

[1]   Centers for Disease Control (CDC). Kaposi's sarcoma and Pneumocystis pneumonia among homosexual men – New York City and California. MMWR 1981; 30(25): 305-8.
[2]   Centers for Disease Control (CDC). Pneumocystis pneumonia – Los Angeles. MMWR 1981; 30(21): 250-2.
[3]   Chesney M. Adherence to HAART Regimens. AIDS Patient Care STDs 2003; 17(4): 169-77.
[4]   Richman DD, Morton SC, Wrin T, *et al*. The prevalence of antiretroviral drug resistance in the United States. AIDS 2004; 18 (10): 1393-401.
[5]   Little SJ, Holte S, Routy RP, *et al*. Antiretroviral-drug resistance among patients recently infected with HIV. N Engl J Med 2002; 347: 385-94.
[6]   Mannheimer SB, Wold N, Gardner EM, *et al*. Mild-to-moderate symptoms during the first year of antiretroviral therapy worsen quality of life in HIV-infected individuals. Clin Infect Dis 2008; 46(6):941-5.
[7]   Strizki J. Targeting HIV attachment and entry for therapy. Adv Pharmacol 2008; 56: 93-120.
[8]   Este JA, Telenti A. HIV entry inhibitors. Lancet 2007; 370(9581): 81-8.
[9]   Horuk R. Chemokine receptor antagonists: overcoming developmental hurdles. Drug Discovery 2009; 8: 23-33.
[10]   Delwart EL, Mosialos G, Gilmore T. Retroviral envelope glycoproteins contain "leucine zipper" like repeat. AIDS Res Hum Retroviruses 1990; 6(6): 703-6.
[11]   Makinson A, Reynes J. The Fusion Inhibitor Enfuvirtide in Recent Antiretroviral Strategies. Current Opin HIV AIDS 2009; 4(2): 150-8.

[12]   Lalezari JP, Enron JJ, Carlson M, *et al*. A Phase II Clinical Study of the Long-Term Safety and Antiviral Activity of Enfuvirtide-Based Antiretroviral Therapy. AIDS 2003; 17(5): 691-8.

[13]   Labross B, Labernardiere JL, Dam E, *et al*. Baseline susceptibility of primary human immunodeficiency Virus Type 1 to Entry Inhibitors. J Virol. 2003; 77(2): 1610-3.

[14]   Zhang X, Nieforth K, Katlama C, *et al*. Pharmacokinetics of Plasma Enfuvirtide After Subcutaneous Administration to Patients with Human Immunodeficiency Virus: Inverse Gaussian Density Absorption and 2-Compartment Disposition. ClinPharmacolTher 2002; 72(1): 10-9.

[15]   Patel IH, Zhang X, Nieforth K, *et al*. Pharmacokinetics, Pharmacodynamics and Drug Interaction Potential of Enfuvirtide. Clinical Pharmacokinetics 2005. 44(2): 175-86.

[16]   Lalezari JP, Patel IH, Zhang X, *et al*. Influence of Subcutaneous Injection Site on the Steady-State Pharmacokinetics of Enfuvirtide (T-20) in HIV-1 Infected Patients. J ClinVirol 2003; 28: 217-22.

[17]   Thompson M, DeJesus EB, Richmond GC, *et al*. Pharmacokinetics, Pharmacodynamics and Safety of Once-Daily *Versus* Twice Daily Dosing with Enfuvirtide in HIV-Infected Subjects. AIDS 2006; 20(3): 397-404.

[18]   Tebas P, Bellos N, Lucasti C, *et al*. Enfuvirtide does not Require Dose Adjustment in Patients with Chronic Kidney Failure: Results of a Pharmacokinetic Study of Enfuvirtide in HIV-1-Infected Patients with Impaired Kidney Function. J Acquir Immune DeficSyndr 2008; 47(3): 342-5.

[19]   Teicher E, Abbara C, Duclos-Vallee JC, *et al*. Enfuvirtide: A Safe and Effective Antiretroviral Agent for Human Immunodeficiency Virus-Infected Patients Shortly After Liver Transplantation. Liver Transpl 2009; 15(10): 1336-42.

[20]   Madeddu G, Calia GM, Campus ML, *et al*. Successful Prevention of Multidrug Resistant HIV Mother-to-Child Transmission with Enfuvirtide Use in Late Pregnancy. Int J STD AIDS 2008; 19(9): 644-5.

[21]   Brennan-Brenson P, Pakianathan M, Rice P, *et al*. Enfuvirtide Prevents Vertical Transmission of Multi-Drug Resistant HIV-1 in Pregnancy But Does Not Cross the Placenta. AIDS 2006; 20(2): 297-9.

[22]   Cohan D, Feakins C, Wara D, *et al*. Perinatal Transmission of Multi-Drug Resistant HIV-1 Despite Viral Suppression on an Enfuvirtide Based Treatment Regimen. AIDS 2005; 19(9): 989-90.

[23]   Myers SA, Selim AA, McDaniel MA, *et al*. A Prospective Clinical and Pathological Examination of Injection Site Reactions with the HIV-1 Fusion Inhibitor Enfuvirtide. AntivirTher 2006; 11(7): 935-9.

[24]   Lalezari JP, Henry K, O'Hearn M, *et al*. Enfuvirtide, an HIV-1 Fusion Inhibitor For Drug-Resistant HIV Infection in North and South America. N Engl J Med 2003; 348(22): 2175-85.

[25]   Lazzarin A, Clotet B, Cooper D, *et al*. Efficacy of Enfuvirtide in Patients Infected with Drug-Resistant HIV-1 in Europe and Australia. N Engl J Med 2003; 348(22): 2186-95.

[26]   Loutfy MR, Antoniou T, Shen S, *et al*. A Large Prospective Study Assessing Injection Site Reactions, Quality of Life and Preference in Patients Using the Biojector *vs* Standard Needles for Enfuvirtide Administration. HIV Med 2007; 8(7): 427-32.

[27]   Lalezari JP, Saag M, Walworth C, *et al*. An Open-Label Safety Study of Enfuvirtide Injection with a Needle-Free Injection Device or Needle/Syringe: the Biojector 2000 Open-Label Safety Study (BOSS). AIDS Res Hum Retroviruses 2008; 24(6) 805-13.

[28]   Allavena C, Prazuck T, Reliquet V, *et al*. Impact of Education and Support on the Tolerability and Quality of Life in a Cohort of HIV-1 Infected Patients Treated with Enfuvirtide (SURCOUF Study). JIAPAC 2008; 4: 187-92.

[29]   Villarroel MC, Martinez E, Riba N, *et al*. Lack of Metabolic Abnormalities and Mitochondrial Toxicity with Enfuvirtide (T-20): A Double-Blind, Placebo-Controlled, Crossover Study with Random Sequence Assignation in Healthy Adult Volunteers. 9th Intl Workshop on Adverse Drug Reactions and Lipodystrophy in HIV 2007 Jul 19-21. Sydney, Australia.

[30]   Zhang X, Lalezari JP, Badley AD, *et al*. Assessment of Drug-Drug Interaction Potential of Enfuvirtide in Human Immunodeficiency Virus Type 1- Infected Patients. ClinPharmacolTher 2004; 75(6): 558-68.

[31]   Boyd M, Ruxrungtham K, Bellibas SE, *et al*. Lack of Interaction between Enfuvirtide and Ritonavir or Ritonavir-Boosted Saquinavir in HIV-1 Infected Patients. J ClinPharmacol 2004; 44(7): 793-802.

[32]   Lu J, Deeks SG, Hoh R, *et al*. Rapid Emergence of Enfuvirtide Resistance in HIV-1 Infected Patients: Results of a Clonal Analysis. J Acquir Immune DeficSyndr 2006; 43(1): 60-4.

[33]   Melby T, Sista P, DeMasi R, *et al*. Characterization of Envelope Glycoprotein gp41 Genotype and Phenotypic Susceptibility to Enfuvirtide at Baseline and on Treatment in the Phase III Clinical Trials TORO1 and TORO2. AIDS Res Hum Retroviruses 2006; 22(5): 375-85.

[34]   Johnson VA, Calvez V, Gunthard HF, *et al*. 2011 Update of the Drug Resistance Mutations in HIV-1. Top Antivir Med 2011; 19(4): 156-64.

[35]   Xu L, Pozniak A, Wildfire A, *et al*. Emergence and Evolution of Enfuvirtide Resistance Following Long Term Therapy Involves Heptad Repeat 2 Mutations Within gp41. Antimicrob Agents Chemother 2005; 49(3): 113-9.

[36]   Wu H, Yao C, Lu RJ. Albuvirtide, the first long-acting HIV fusion inhibitor, suppressed viral replication in HIV-infected adults [abstract H-554]. Proceedings of the 52nd Interscience Conference on Antimicrobials and Chemotherapy (ICAAC). September 9-12, 2012. San Francisco. .

[37]   Chong H, Yao X, Zhang C, *et al*. Biophysical property and broad anti-HIV activity of albuvirtide, a 3-maleimimidopropionic acid-modified peptide fusion inhibitor. PLoS One 2012; 7(3):e32599.

[38]   Moyle GJ, Wildfire A, Mandalia S, *et al*. Epidemiology and predictive factors for chemokine receptor use in HIV-1 infection. J Infect Dis 2005 Mar 15; 191(6):866-72.

[39]   Melby T, Despirito M, Demasi R, *et al*. HIV-1 coreceptor use in triple-class treatment-experienced patients: baseline prevalence, correlates, and relationship to enfuvirtide response. J Infect Dis 2006 Jul 15; 194(2):238-46.

[40]   Trinh L, Han D, Huang W, *et al*. Technical validation of an enhanced sensitivity *Trofile* HIV coreceptor tropism assay for selecting patients for therapy with entry inhibitors targeting CCR5. Antiviral Ther 2008; 13:A128.

[41]   Reeves J Han D, Liu Y, *et al*. Enhancements to the *Trofile* HIV coreceptor tropism assay enable reliable detection of CXCR4-using subpopulations at less than 1% [abstract]. Proceedings of the 47th Interscience Conference on Antimicrobial Agents and Chemotherapy; September 17-20, 2007; Chicago, Illinois.

[42]   Vandekerckhove LP, Wensing AM, Kaiser R, *et al*. European guidelines on the clinical management of HIV-1 tropism testing. Lancet Infect Dis 2011 May; 11(5):394-407.

[43]   Wilkin TJ, Goetz MB, Leduc R, *et al*. Reanalysis of coreceptor tropism in HIV-1-infected adults using a phenotypic assay with enhanced sensitivity. Clin Infect Dis 2011; 52(7): 925-8.

[44]   Nichols WG, Steel HM, Bonny T, *et al*. Hepatotoxicity observed in clinical trials of aplaviroc (GW873140). Antimicrob Agents Chemother 2008; 52(3): 858-65.

[45]   Abel S, van der Ryst E, Rosario MC, *et al*. Assessment of the pharmacokinetics, safety and tolerability of maraviroc, a novel CCR5 antagonist, in healthy volunteers. Br J ClinPharmacol 2008; 65(S1): 5-18.

[46]   Selzentry (maraviroc) [package insert]. Triangle Park, NC: Viiv Healthcare, 2013.

[47]   Dumond JB, Patterson KB, Pecha AL, *et al*. Maraviroc concentrates in the cervicovaginal fluid and vaginal tissue of HIV-negative women. J Acquir Immune DeficSyndr 2009; 51(15): 546-53.

[48]   Tiraboschi JM, Curto J, Niubo J, *et al*. Maraviroc levels in cerebrospinal fluid (CSF) and seminal plasma from HIV-infected patients [abstract plus poster no.114]. Proceedings of the 17th Conference on Retroviruses and Opportunistic Infections; 2010 Feb 16-19; San Francisco, CA, USA.

[49]   Brown K, Patterson K, Malone S, *et al*. Antiretrovirals for prevention: maraviroc exposure in the semen and rectal tissue of healthy male volunteers after single and multiple dosing [abstract no. 85]. 17th Conference on Retroviruses and Opportunistic Infections; 2010 Feb 16-19; San Francisco, CA, USA.

[50]   Panel of Treatment of HIV-Infected Pregnant Women and Prevention of Perinatal Transmission. Perinatal HIV Guidelines Working Group Members. Recommendations for the use of antiretroviral drugs in pregnant HIV-1-infected women for maternal health and interventions to reduce perinatal HIV transmission in the United States. Retrieved February 17, 2013. Available on the World Wide Web at: http://aidsinfo.nih.gov/

[51]   Johnson AA, Ray AS, Hanes J, *et al*. Toxicity of antiviral nucleoside analogs and the human mitochondrial DNA polymerase. J Biol Chem 2001; 276(44): 40847-40857.

[52]   Bierman WF, van Agtmael MA, Nijhuis M, *et al*. HIV monotherapy with ritonavir-boosted protease inhibitors: a systematic review. AIDS 2009; 23(3): 279-291.

[53]   Mills A, Mildvan D, Podzamczer D, *et al*. Once-daily maraviroc in combination with ritonavir-boosted atazanavir in treatment naïve patients infected with CCR5-tropic HIV-1 (study A400108):

96-week results. [abstract tuab0102] XIX International AIDS Conference. 2012 Jul 22-27; Washington DC, USA.

[54] Taiwo B, Swindells S, Berzins B, *et al.* Week 48 results of the Maraviroc Plus Darunavir/ritonavir Study (MIDAS) for treatment naïve patients infected with R5-tropic HIV-1. [abstract tupe099] XIX International AIDS Conference. 2012 Jul 22-27; Washington DC, USA.

[55] Taylor S, Arribas J, Perno CF, *et al.* Efficacy of maraviroc (MVC) administered once or twice daily with boosted protease inhibitors to treatment experienced patients. [Abstract tuab0106] 6th IAS Conference on HIV Pathogenesis, Treatment and Prevention. 2011 Jul 17-20; Rome, Italy.

[56] Abel S, Davis JD, Ridgeway CE, *et al.* Pharmacokinetics, safety and tolerability of a single dose of maraviroc in HIV-negative subjects with mild or moderate hepatic impairment. Antiviral Therapy 2009; 14(6): 831-7.

[57] MacInnes A, Lazzarin A, Di Perri G, *et al.* Maraviroc can improve lipid profiles in dyslipidemic patients with HIV: results from the MERIT trial. HIV Clin Trials 2011; 12(1): 24-36.

[58] Hyland R, Dickins M, Collins C, *et al.* Maraviroc: *in vitro* assessment of drug-drug interaction potential. Br J ClinPharmacol 2008; 66(4): 498-507.

[59] Abel S, Jenkins TM, Whitlock LA, *et al.* Effects of CYP3A4 inducers with and without CYP3A4 inhibitors on the pharmacokinetics of maraviroc in healthy volunteers. Br J ClinPharmacol 2008; 65(S1): 38-46

[60] Abel S, Russell D, Taylor-Worth RJ, *et al.* Effects of CYP 3A4 inhibitors on the pharamcokinetics of maraviroc in healthy volunteers. Br J ClinPharmacol 2008; 65(S1): 27-37.

[61] Abel S, Russell D, Whitlock LA, *et al.* The effects of cotrimoxazole or tenofovir co-administration on the pharmacokinetics of maraviroc in healthy volunteers. Br J ClinPharmacol 2008; 65(S1): 47-53.

[62] AbelS, Russel D, Whitlock LA, *et al.* Effect of maraviroc on the pharmacokinetics of midazolam, lamivudine/zidovudine, and ethinylestradiol/levonorgestrel in healthy volunteers. Br J ClinPharmacol 2008; 65(S1): 19-26.

[63] Andrews E, Glue P, Fang J, *et al.* Assessment of the pharmacokinetics of co-administered maraviroc and raltegravir. Br J ClinPharmacol 2010; 69(1): 51-7.

[64] Gulick RM, Lalezari J, Goodrich J, *et al.* Maraviroc for Previously Treated Patients with R5 HIV-1 Infection. N Engl J Med 2008; 359(14): 1429-41.

[65] Hardy WD, Gulick RM, Mayer H, *et al.* Two-year safety and virologic efficacy of maraviroc in treatment-experienced patients with CCR5-tropic HIV-1 Infection: 96-week combined analysis of MOTIVATE 1 and 2. J Acquir Immune DeficSyndr 2010; 55(5): 558-564.

[66] Cooper DA, Heera J, Goodrich J, *et al.* Maraviroc *versus* Efavirenz, both in combination with zidovudine-lamivudine, for the treatment of antiretroviral-naïve subjects with CCR5-tropic HIV-1 infection. J Infect Dis 2010; 201: 803-13.

[67] Sierra-Madero J, Di Perri G, Wood R, *et al.* Efficacy and Safety of Maraviroc *Versus* Efavirenz, both with zidovudine/lamivudine: 96-week results from the MERIT Study. HIV Clin Trials 2010; 11(3): 125-32.

[68] Swenson LC, Mo T, Dong WWY, *et al.* Deep V3 Sequencing for HIV Type 1 Tropism in Treatment Naïve Patients: A Reanalysis of the MERIT Trial of Maraviroc. Clin Infect Dis 2011; 53: 732-42.

[69] National Institute of Allergy and Infectious Diseases. Evaluating the safety and tolerability of antiretroviral drug regimens used as pre-exposure prophylaxis to prevent HIV infection in at-risk men who have sex with men and in at-risk women. In: ClinicalTrials.gov [Internet]. Bethesda (MD): National Library of Medicine (US). 2000- [cited 2014 Mar 12]. Available from http://clinicaltrials.gov/ct2/show/NCT01505114/_NLM Identifier: NCT01505114.

[70] Brown KC, Patterson KB, Malone SA, *et al.* Single and multiple dose pharmacokinetics of maraviroc in saliva, semen, and rectal tissue of healthy HIV-negative men. Journal of Infectious Diseases 2011; 203 (10): 1484-1490.

[71] Dummond JB, Patterson KB, Pecha AL, *et al.* Maraviroc concentrates in the cervicovaginal fluid and vaginal tissue of HIV-negative women. Journal of Acquired Immunodeficiency Syndromes 2009; 51(5): 546-553.

[72] McGovern RA, Thielen A, Mo T, *et al.* Population-based V3 genotypic tropism assay: a retrospective analysis using screening samples from the A4001029 and MOTIVATE studies. AIDS 2010; 24: 2517-25.

[73] Westby M. Resistance to CCR5 Antagonists. CurrOpin HIV AIDS 2007; 2(2): 137-44.

[74]   Moore JP, Kuritzkes DR. A piece de resistance: how HIV-1 escapes small molecule CCR5 inhibitors. CurrOpin HIV AIDS 2009; 4(2): 118-24.
[75]   Ratcliff AN, Shi W, Arts EJ. HIV-1 resistance to maraviroc conferred by a CD4 binding site mutation in the envelope glycoprotein gp120. J Virol 2013; 87(2): 923-34.

CHAPTER 3

Reverse Transcriptase Inhibitors

Amy Moss[1], Cara Felton[2] and Sarah Nanzigu[3],*

[1]*Thomas Street Health Center, Harris Health System, Houston, TX, USA;* [2]*School of Pharmacy and Pharmaceutical Sciences, University at Buffalo, Buffalo, NY, USA* and [3]*Department of Pharmacology and Therapeutics, Makerere University College of Health Sciences, Uganda*

Abstract: The first revelation of HIV belonging to retroviruses with its genetic material stored as RNA indicated its need for reverse transcription as one of the steps in its lifecycle. This opened the way to the therapeutic battle against the virus. Reverse transcriptase inhibitors are the oldest antiretroviral agents inhibiting the formation of viral DNA from RNA. Some of these agents work as analogues of the naturally occurring nucleoside and nucleotide bases required for DNA formation, hence their insertion into a growing DNA chain leads to its termination. Another group does not mimic natural DNA bases but rather bind to and disfigure the reverse transcriptase enzyme. The former are referred to as nucleoside and nucleotide reverse transcriptase Inhibitors (NRTI), while the later are non-nucleoside reverse transcriptase inhibitors (NNRTI). These agents are used in combination with other antiretroviral agents, and some of them have activity against hepatitis B which is a common HIV co-infection.

Keywords: Reverse Transcriptase Inhibitors, RTI, NRTI, NNRTI, Antiretroviral Drugs, HIV, ART, Tenofovir, Efavirenz, Emtricitabine, Etravirine, Rilpivirine, Zidovudine.

GENERAL INTRODUCTION

Historically, treatment regimens evolved from the use of one or two nucleoside reverse transcriptase inhibitors (NRTIs) to a combination of two NRTIs plus a third antiretroviral agent. Combination therapy with 3-to-4 NRTIs demonstrated antiviral activity but either lack comparable data with other regimens or were shown to be inferior to other combination regimens [1]. As most of the clinical trials data have been based on the use of 2 NRTIs, the current strategy for most treatment regimens recommended by the treatment guidelines consists of 2 NRTIs with a third agent from a different class. Although this has been used with success for almost two decades, a new research may lead to a different approach with class-sparing

Corresponding author Sarah Nanzigu: Department of Pharmacology and Therapeutics, Makerere University College of Health Sciences, Kampala, Uganda; Tel: 256784843045; Fax: 256414532947; E-mails: snanzigu@yahoo.com; snanzigu@chs.mak.ac.ug

regimens (*i.e.* reservation of a particular class of drugs in order to avoid toxicities and viral resistance while maintaining maximal viral suppression) [2].

Recommendations for antiretroviral regimens are similar among the DHHS guidelines and IAS-USA guidelines as well as the British and European guidelines [3-6]. The differences in the recommended agents are again largely based on differing interpretations of clinical data. All of these combination regimens have been demonstrated to be efficacious. However, it should be noted that every individual antiretroviral agent and every regimen have different pharmacokinetic profiles, drug-drug interactions, side effects and toxicities. The optimal choice of agents for a regimen is dependent on the specific needs, situation and co-morbidities of the individual that is being treated. The critical issues to consider are adherence barriers/lifestyle (*i.e.*, once *vs.* twice daily, need for co-administration with food, co-formulated agents), co-morbidities (*i.e.*, hepatitis B, pregnancy, kidney disease), and tolerability (side effects that the patient can tolerate). The successful regimen will usually be the regimen that is well –tolerated and is well suited for the individual's lifestyle.

The recommendation to use 2 NRTIs in combination with one or two agents from another class gives room to employing regimens that constitute agents from reverse transcriptase inhibitors (RTI) class only [7, 8]. Moreover, such combinations are more available and affordable in resource limited settings. This pronounces the importance of the enzyme reverse transcriptase as a target in the fight against HIV/AIDS. The development of the first ever approved antiretroviral agent Zidovudine and related agents followed a revelation that HIV was a retrovirus hence uses the reverse transcriptase enzyme to form its DNA [9, 10]. Among the drugs targeting this enzyme are some that mimic its substrates (nucleoside and nucleotide analogues) and those that do not look like the substrates but are able to attack and denature the activity of the enzyme (non-nucleosides). They are classified into nucleoside or nucleotide reverse transcriptase inhibitors (NRTIs); and non-nucleoside reverse transcriptase inhibitors (NNRTIs).

THE NUCLEOSIDE REVERSE TRANCRIPTASE INHIBITORS

NRTIs inhibit the virally-encoded reverse transcriptase enzyme in the host cell cytoplasm. This blocks the conversion of viral single-stranded RNA to double-stranded DNA, ultimately preventing incorporation of HIV genetic material into the host genome. NRTIs mimic nucleoside bases (cytidine, uridine, adenosine, guanosine, thymidine and inosine), that are required during the formation of DNA

[11]. The nucleoside analogues compete with natural nucleosides, and when reverse transcriptase incorporates them into the growing DNA chain, elongation is halted (Fig. **1**). First NRTIs must first be activated in the cell through three phosphorylation steps before they can become active chain terminators. NRTIs are poor substrates for nuclear DNA polymerases, but some NRTIs are utilized by mitochondrial polymerases, hence explaining some of the side effects during NRTI use [11].

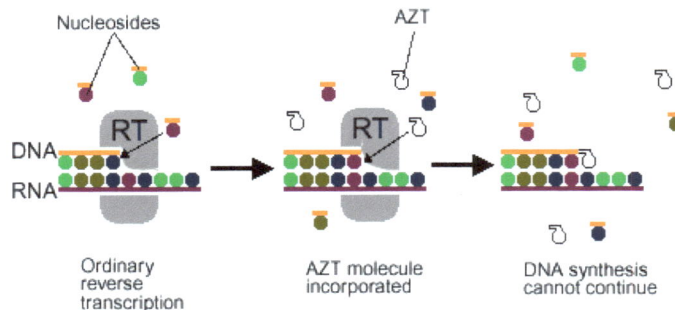

Fig. (1). Illustration of the mode of action of nucleoside reverse transcriptase inhibitors.

PHARMACOLOGY OF NRTIs

Similarity is observed in the pharmacology of reverse transcriptase inhibitors falling under the same category-nucleosides, nucleotides and non-nucleosides. Therefore, modes of action and toxicity profiles often characterize categories of drugs shown in Tables **1-3**.

Zidovudine; Azidothymidine, AZT

Zidovudine was the first breakthrough in HIV therapy, registered by FDA in 1986 [12]. Azidothymidine (AZT) is an anologue of thymidine where the 3´hydroxyl group of thymidine is replaced by an azido group. AZT was first prepared as an anticancer agent in 1964 which did not show the required efficacy against cancer, but the drug was later reported to have activity against retroviruses. Key pharmacology parameters of AZT are summarized in Appendix **1** (Table **5**).

Emtricitabine, FTC (Emtriva)

Emtricitabine is a synthetic nucleoside analog of cytidine. Following three steps of phosphorylation, emtricitabine 5'-triphosphate competes with the natural substrate deoxycytidine 5'-triphosphate and its incorporation into nascent viral DNA results in chain termination. Emtricitabine was first approved by the FDA in July 2003 for use in HIV infected persons aged 18 years and above, but expanded to cover other groups. It is available on market as a single 200mg capsule, an oral 10 mg/mL solution and co-formulated tablets containing 300 mg of tenofovir disoproxil fumarate and 200 mg of emtricitabine (truvada), or 300mg Tenofovir+ 200mg Emtricitabine+ 600mg Efavirenz. Emtricitabine in combination with tenofovir are currently regarded to form a strong backbone for first line therapy against HIV. The recommended dose for adults is 200mg once a day, and children receive 6-mg/kg dose, up to a maximum of 200 mg [13, 14].

Table 1. List and availability of approved drugs NRTIs.

Brand Name	Generic Name	Manufacturer Name	Approval Date (dd-mmm-yy)
Combivir	lamivudine and zidovudine	GlaxoSmithKline	27-Sep-97
Emtriva	emtricitabine, FTC	Gilead Sciences	02-Jul-03
Epivir	lamivudine, 3TC	GlaxoSmithKline	17-Nov-95
Epzicom	abacavir and lamivudine	GlaxoSmithKline	02-Aug-04
Hivid	zalcitabine, dideoxycytidine, ddC (no longer marketed)	Hoffmann-La Roche	19-Jun-92
Retrovir	zidovudine, azidothymidine, AZT, ZDV	GlaxoSmithKline	19-Mar-87
Trizivir	abacavir, zidovudine, and lamivudine	GlaxoSmithKline	14-Nov-00
Videx EC	enteric coated didanosine, ddI EC	Bristol Myers-Squibb	31-Oct-00
Videx	didanosine, dideoxyinosine, ddI	Bristol Myers-Squibb	9-Oct-91
Zerit	stavudine, d4T	Bristol Myers-Squibb	24-Jun-94
Ziagen	abacavir sulfate, ABC	GlaxoSmithKline	17-Dec-98

Antiretroviral drugs used in the treatment of HIV infection. [Page Last Updated: 12/18/2012] http://www.fda.gov/ForConsumers/byAudience/ForPatientAdvocates/HIVandAIDSActivities/ucm118915.htm

Pharmacokinetics and Pharmacogenetics

Emtricitabine is well absorbed following the oral route, leading to bioavailability of up to 93%. The adult 200mg and pediatric 6mg/kg doses produce a median area under the curve (AUC) of approximately 10 h*µg/ml; maximum concentration (C_{max}) of 1.8 ± 0.7 µg/ml and minimum concentrations (C_{min}) of 0.09 ± 0.07 µg/ml [13, 14]. Emtricitabine undergoes glomerular filtration and active tubular secretion, with limited amount undergoing oxidation and conjugation in the liver. Its terminal half-life is estimated at 10 hours. Significant drug interactions may occur with inhibitors of organic ion, organic cation and nucleoside transport inhibitors including trimethoprim [15]. Reduced renal clearance has been observed in patients taking emtricitabine in combination with tenofovir, and the drug should be avoided if creatinine clearance (Cr) is below 50mL/min [15]. The exposure of emtricitabine is about 25% lower during pregnancy; however, these levels are adequate for viral suppression, including reducing the risk of mother to child transmission [16].

Lactic acidosis and hepatomegaly with steatosis are common toxicities in NRTIs. Summary of key pharmacokinetic characteristics for additional nucleoside reverse transcriptase inhibitors are listed in appendix **1**.

THE NUCLEOTIDE REVERSE TRANSCRIPTASE INHIBITORS

Nucleotide reverse transcriptase inhibitors (NtRTIs) are analogues of natural nucleotides (cytidine monophosphate, uridine monophosphate, adenosine monophosphate, guanosine monophosphate, deoxythymidine monophosphate and inosine monophosphate). Their mechanism of action is similar to nucleoside reverse transcriptase inhibitors; however, since NtRTI compounds are monophosphorylated, therefore they require only two enzymatic reactions to become active moieties [11]. Tenofovir DF is currently the only NtRTI approved by the U.S. Food and Drug Administration (FDA) for HIV treatment.

Table 2. List and availability of approved drugs NtRTI.

Truvada	Tenofovir disoproxil fumarate and emtricitabine	Gilead Sciences, Inc.	02-Aug-04
Viread	Tenofovir disoproxil fumarate, TDF	Gilead	26-Oct-01

Antiretroviral drugs used in the treatment of HIV infection. [Page Last Updated: 12/18/2012] http://www.fda.gov/ForConsumers/byAudience/ForPatientAdvocates/HIVandAIDSActivities/ucm118915.htm

PHARMACOLOGY OF NtRTIs

Tenofovir

Tenofovir-diphosphate is an analogue of the natural 2'-deoxyadenosine-triphosphate. The mode of action is similar to all NRTIs. Tenofovir is a monophosphate analogue and therefore requires diphosphorylation to become active [11]. Tenofovir is polar and ionized which makes it to be poorly absorbed, while its pro-drug disoproxil di-ester masks the non-polar regions enhancing its absorption [11]. The oral bioavailability of a 300-mg dose of tenofovir disoproxil fumarate is approximately 25%, and increased after a fat diet, with the AUC and C_{max} increased by 40% and 14%, respectively [11]. Administration with food is therefore advised. The median peak concentration of tenofovir with food is 326 ng/ml and AUC is 3324 ng hour/ml. Tenofovir diphosphate undergoes active tubular secretion with OAT-1 and OAT-3 as the main renal transporters [11].

The plasma half-life of tenofovir is 17hour but the triphosphate form is ionized and trapped intracellularly prolonging its half-life to 150 hours. The intracellular half-lives of both tenofovir-DP and emtricitabine-TP are the longest for the NRTI class, making them pharmacologically favorable for pre-exposure prophylaxis [11]. Tenofovir gives a dose and concentration dependent reduction for the risk of HIV-1 infection. The lowest level of reduction is at 76% following two doses of tenofovir taken weekly, and the observed maximum reduction is 99% at seven doses of tenofovir every week [11].

Toxicity

The main toxicity concern for tenofovir is damage of proximal renal tubule due to accumulation of tenofovir following the organic anion transporter OAT-1 and OAT-3 uptake of the drug into the cells [11].

THE NON-NUCLEOSIDE REVERSE TRANSCRIPTASE INHIBITORS

Table 3. List and availability of approved drugs NNRTIs.

Brand Name	Generic Name	Manufacturer Name	Approval Date (dd-mmm-yy)
Edurant	Rilpivirine	Tibotec Therapeutics	20-May-11
Intelence	Etravirine	Tibotec Therapeutics	18-Jan-08
Rescriptor	Delavirdine, DLV	Pfizer	4-Apr-97
Sustiva	Efavirenz, EFV	Bristol Myers-Squibb	17-Sep-98
Viramune (Immediate Release)	Nevirapine, NVP	Boehringer Ingelheim	21-Jun-96
Viramune XR (Extended Release)	Nevirapine, NVP	Boehringer Ingelheim	25-Mar-11

Antiretroviral drugs used in the treatment of HIV infection. [Page Last Updated: 12/18/2012] http://www.fda.gov/ForConsumers/byAudience/ForPatientAdvocates/HIVandAIDSActivities/ucm118915.htm

NNRTIs also inhibit reverse transcriptase in the cytoplasm of the host cell. They act at the same point in the HIV-1 replication cycle as do the NRTIs, but NNRTIs bind the reverse transcriptase adjacent to the active site, causing structural alterations, and disruption of the enzyme's catalytic site, hence preventing it from adding any new nucleosides to the growing DNA chain. Because of this difference in mechanism of action, the viral mutations that encode for NNRTIs resistance differ from those for NRTIs resistance. NNRTIs are characterised with long half-lives and are largely metabolised by CYP450 enzymes, mainly the CYP3A4 and CYP2B6, with some of the agents having the ability to induce or inhibit these enzymes [17, 18].

PHARMACOLOGY OF APPROVED NNRTIs

Efavirenz

Efavirenz and other NNRTIs- nevirapine, delavirdine, etravirine and rilpivirine- are not analogues of the naturally occuring nucleosides, they do not require intracellular phosphorylation to become active, and neither do they interfere with this process [19, 20]. Efavirenz is the most widely used NNRTI, and current FDA recommendations for its use include treatment of HIV-1 infected adults and pediatric patients at least 3 months old and weighing at least 3.5 kg [3, 21].

Pharmacokinetics and Pharmacogenetics

Efavirenz has a low bioavailability of 40-45%, increased by fat diet, and reduced in some disease conditions, including HIV [22-24]. Formulations to enhance drug bioavailability are under investigation, including the Solid lipid nanoparticle (SLN) formulations that have been shown to significantly improve the oral bioavailability of Efavirenz, and reduces the interindividual variability in plasma concentrations [23, 25, 26]. The half-life of Efavirenz is about 72 hours following a single dose, but reduces to 40-55 hours with repeated administration, owing to auto-induction [20, 21, 27]. Efavirenz, is mainly catalysed by CYP2B6, assisted by CYP3A5, CYP1A2 and CYP3A4 [28, 29]. The action of additional enzymes; CYP2A6, CYP2C19 is observed at increasing efavirenz concentrations [28, 29]. The primary and major metabolite of Efavirenz is 8-hydroxyefavirenz, which may subsequently be hydroxylated to 8, 14-dihydroxyefavirenz, and 7-hydroxyefavirenz is a minor metabolite [29-31]. Efavirenz is also a substrate of the P-glycoprotein, and may also undergo glucuronodisation, primarily by UGT2B7, with subsequent polymorphisms contributing to variation in efavirenz exposure [32-35]. Efavirenz shows a gene-dependant induction of the activity of enzymes responsible for its own metabolism, with fast metabolising genotypes exerting a more extensive enzyme induction [34, 36-42]. The auto-induction phenomenon is due to the drugs' strong ability to activate the human constitutive androgenic receptor (hCAR) and human pregnane X receptor (hPXR) that are key transcription regulators of the CYP2B6 and CY3A4 [36, 43]. The activation of these receptors lead to: gene, time and dose dependant induction of the CYP2B6 and 3A4 enzymes, resulting into intra and interindividual variation in efavirenz exposure

[27, 39, 40, 44, 45]. Notably, CYP26*6 genotype is associated with reduced enzyme activity which result into reduced efavirenz clearence, and a resultant increase in plasma concentrations [35, 46-49]. The genotype is more prevalent among African populations, and persons of Papa New Guinea origin, with recent data suggesting efavirenz dose reduction for these populations [39, 50-52]. Efavirenz also induces CYP2C19, CYP3A5, UGT2B7, and ABCB1 [18, 34, 38-40]. The effect of efavirenz on CYP3A4 and 2C19 may be mixed with instances of initial inhibition followed by induction. Efavirenz also has minimal inhibition of CYP1A2, 2C9 and 2D6 [18, 53]. Efavirenz has also been observed to up-regulate several drug transporters including ABCB and SLCO groups of transporter [54]. The ability of efavirenz to induce activity of metaolising enzymes has several clinically relevant drug-interactions that are discussed in chapter 7 of this book.

Toxicity

The most common unwanted effects experienced during Efavirenz-based antiretroviral therapy, are neuropsychiatric disorders that include: sleep disorders, mood changes and fatigue [55, 56]. The neuropsychiatric disorders are observed early in the course of Efavirenz/Nevirapine based therapy, and relate to genotype and drug concentrations [27, 57, 58]. Usually, the symptoms are mild-moderate and transient, although some may persist to one or two years, and severe cases including suicidality and/or status epilepticus have also been reported [56, 59, 60]. Neuropsychiatric events have been reported in about 10% of the Caucasian patient population, but the prevalence is much higher in people of the African origin [27, 55]. Liver toxicity has been reported in some patients using efavirenz, but the risk for occurrence and the degree of severity is much higher with Nevirapine use [41, 61]. Dermatological and gastrointestinal disorders may also occur in up to 3 % of the patient population [55].

Drug Resistance

Resistance to efavirenz follows mutations within HIV-1 Reverse Transcriptase gene, and most resistance genes can be transmitted to other drugs in the NNRTI class [62-65]. All NNRTIs have a low barrier to resistance, with one mutation, including minority drug resistance mutations being sufficient to confer resistance that reduces drug efficacy [66, 67]. K103N is the major mutation that confers resistance to NNRTIs, and others include: T215Y, M41L, L100I, V108I, Y188L, G190S, and P225H [62, 63, 66-69]. With the exception of Y181C mutation that confers resistance to Nevirapine and not efavirenz, the above resistance mutations during therapy with a NNRTI would be selected by other drugs in the same class [63, 64, 70].

Rilpivirine RPV (Edurant)

DHHS guidelines have recommended RPV as an alternate regimen. Approval of Rilpivirine was based on two Phase 3 studies, ECHO and THRIVE. In a pooled analysis of ECHO and THRIVE, a total of 1368 patients were randomized across the two studies (n= 690 in ECHO, n=678 in THRIVE) [71]. In the pooled analysis, a lower incidence of grade 2-4 adverse events and rate of discontinuations due to adverse events were observed in the Rilpivirine arm compared to the efavirenz arm. Additionally, there were lower rates of dizziness, abnormal dreams/ nightmares and rash observed in the Rilpivirine arm *vs.* efavirenz arm [71]. Depressive disorders (depressed mood, depression, dysphoria, major depression, mood altered, negative thoughts, suicide attempts, suicidal ideation) regardless of causality or severity was 8% with RPV and 6% with EFV. Most events were mild or moderate in severity. Grade 3 or 4 events were 1% in each arm. Suicide was reported in two patients on RPV; suicide ideation was reported in 1 patient on RPV and 3 patients on EFV [72]. Baseline lipid parameters were similar between both groups at baseline. Treatment emergent lipid abnormalities occurred at a significantly higher incidence in the EFV group than in the Rilpivirine arm. Rilprivirine is mainly metabolized by CY3A4, CYP2C19, CYP1A2, and it is a weak inducer of CYP3A4, CYP2B6 and 2C19 [18, 65].

Etravirine, ETR (Intelence[®])

Etravirine is a di-aryl-pyrimidine (DAPY) derivative non-nucleoside reverse transcriptase inhibitor (NNRTI), and has activity against HIV-1 by binding to reverse transcriptase. It blocks the RNA-dependent and DNA-dependent DNA polymerase activities, including HIV-1 replication. The inherent molecular flexibility of ETR relative to other NNRTIs permits the compound to retain its binding affinity to the reverse transcriptase despite the changes induced by common NNRTI resistance mutations [73].

Dose Recommendations

Usual dosing recommendation in adults is Etravirine 200 mg, by mouth, twice daily, with food.[2] Etravirine is not recommended for children and adolescents less than 6 years of age or less than 16 kilograms (kg), as use has not been evaluated. Dose is weight based and 25 mg tablets are available for children 6–18 years old, given according to the information in Table **4** [73, 74]. No dosage adjustments have been suggested in renal or hepatic impairment.

Table 4. Dosage recommendations for Etravirine in children and adolescents.

Children and adolescents ≥6 years	Dosing Recommendation
16 to <20 kg	100 mg twice daily
20 to <25 kg	125 mg twice daily
25 to <30 kg	150 mg twice daily
≥30 kg	200 mg twice daily

Tablets can be dissolved in 5 mL of water and taken with orange juice or milk, if desired. Dissolved tablets should be taken immediately and completely. Grapefruit juice and warm (over 104° F) or carbonated beverages should be avoided [74].

Pharmacokinetics of Etravirine in Adult Patients

In healthy volunteer studies Etravirine administration demonstrated dose-proportional kinetics [73].

__Maximum Concentrations (C_{max}):__ Treatment-experienced HIV-1-infected adults receiving ETR PO 200 mg twice daily for 48 weeks resulted in C_{max} of 297 +/- 391 ng/mL, (median: 298 ng/mL; range: 2 to 4852 ng/mL) [73]. Peak concentration in 8 HIV-1-infected adults following ETR PO 400 mg once daily for 7 days was 704 ng /mL (range, 470 to 1510 ng/mL). Despite C_{max} being 76 % greater when 400mg ETR was administered once daily compared to 200mg twice daily, there was no significant difference in intracellular concentrations (mean Cmax 1.23 (90% CI, 0.89 to 1.7) [75]. Time to Peak Concentration (T_{max}) is approximately 2.5 to 4 hours [73].

__Area Under the Curve (AUC):__ In treatment-experienced HIV-1-infected adults receiving ETR PO 200 mg twice daily for 48 weeks the AUC (0 to 12 hours) resulted in the following; mean: 4522 +/- 4710 ng x hr/mL; median: 4380 ng x hr/mL; and range: 458 to 59,084 ng x hr/mL [73]. In the 8 HIV-1-infected adults that received ETR PO 400 mg once daily for 7 days the AUC was 30 % greater (mean: 9119 ng x hr/mL and range: 5559 to 22,946 ng x hr/mL), but intracellular concentrations were not significantly different [75].

CSF (% of serum): The 2010 CNS Penetration Effectiveness (CPE) score of ETR is 2 out of 4, and this ranking strongly predicts HIV-1 replication in CSF when viral replication is suppressed in the plasma [76].

Protein Binding

Etravirine is highly protein bound (>99.8%) to albumin (99.6%) and alpha 1-acid glycoprotein (97.66% to 99.02%) [73].

Effect of Food on the Pharmacokinetics of Etravirine

Etravirine should be taken with food because a standard breakfast boosts the AUC by 51% compared to a fasted state. Clinically significant differences in AUC have not been demonstrated with various types of food [77].

Metabolism and Elimination

Etravirine is a substrate of CYP3A4, CYP2C9, and CYP2C19, a weak inducer of CYP3A4, a weak inhibitor of CYP2C9, and a moderate inhibitor of CYP2C19, and p-glycoprotein [73]. Mean elimination half-life of ETR is approximately 41 (+/- 20) hours [73]. Minimal loss of Etravirine occurs during dialysis owing to the fact that ETR is heavily protein bound, and hence dosage adjustment may not be required in renal impairment [73, 78]

Pharmacokinetics in Pediatric Patients

A population pharmacokinetic model by kakuda *et al.*, indicates that Etravirine 5.2mg/kg BID in children and adolescents (6-17 years) provides comparable exposure to adults receiving 200mg BID [79].

Effect of Sex, Body Weight, Age, and Race on Pharmacokinetics

Pharmacokinetics of Etravirine are not affected by sex and race, but a trend for higher ETR levels was demonstrated with increased age as well as decreased weight in HIV-1 infected patients [80].

Pharmacokinetics in Pregnant Women

Etravirine is a Pregnancy Category B and should be utilized during pregnancy only if the potential benefit justifies the potential risk, as ETR crosses the placenta barrier [81]. Case series by Izureita *et al.*, where PK of ETR was assessments in 5 pregnant women showed that concentrations in the 3rd trimester are comparable to those seen in non-pregnant adults. Therefore, dosage adjustment are not required during pregnancy [82]. Excretion of ETR in breast milk is unknown, but complete avoidance of breast-feeding by HIV-infected women, in the United States, is recommended to decrease the potential for HIV transmission [81].

Adverse Events

The most common side effects for Etravirine include rash and peripheral neuropathy. While rash is a class-wide adverse effect of currently approved NNRTIs, lower rates of rash and central nervous system adverse events have been observed with ETR compared to other NNRTIs [83]. If a rash develops from Etravirine, then the FDA advises to discontinue immediately, but it may be possible to tolerate another NNRTI [74].

Additional Warnings and Precautions

Additional warnings related to adverse effects include, fat redistribution, immune reconstitution syndrome, and skin reactions or hypersensitivity (usually occurs during second week of initiation) [73].

Drug Interactions

Etravirine is a potent inducer of CYP3A4, metabolized by CYP3A4 and CYP2C, and inhibits CYP2C, 2C19 and p- glycoprotein. High potential for interactions exist because of substantial involvement with the CYP 450 enzymes [73].

Enzyme Action:	Effect if Co-administered:
ETR induces CYP3A4	↓ plasma levels of drugs metabolized by CYP3A4
ETR inhibits CYP2C, 2C19, and p-glycoprotein	↑ plasma levels of drugs metabolized by CYP2C, 2C19, and p-glycoprotein
Substrates of CYP3A4, CYP2C9, CYP2C19 and/or p-glycoprotein	May alter the therapeutic effect or adverse reaction profile of the co- administered drugs
Drugs that inhibit CYP3A4 or CYP2C	↑ Etravirine plasma levels
Drugs that induce CYP3A4 or CYP2C	↓ Etravirine plasma levels
Inhibitors or inducers of CYP3A4, CYP2C9, and/or CYP2C19	May alter the therapeutic effect or adverse reaction profile of Etravirine

Avoid co-administration of ETR with other NNRTIs, and ritonavir boosted protease inhibitors except Daurnavir/Ritonavir or Kaletra [73, 74]. Co-administered Maraviroc may require dose adjustment depending on whether the additional ARVs in the patient's regimen affect the pharmacokinetics of Maraviroc [73, 74]. Other drugs to be avoided during ETR use include carbamazepine, phenobarbital, phenytoin, Rifapentine, or rifampin while antifungal agents, lipid lowering drugs, warfarin and diazepam can be used with caution [73, 74].

Resistance

Seventeen mutations associated with decreased virological response to Etravirine have been identified. These include, in order of weighted score for resistance, Y181I, Y181V, K101P, L100I, Y181C, 230L, 138A, V106I, G190S, V179F, V90I, A98G, K101E, 101H, 138G, 138K, 138Q, V179D, 179T and G190A. At least 3 must be present before Etravirine response is equivalent to placebo [84].

CONFLICT OF INTEREST

The authors confirm that this chapter contents have no conflict of interest.

ACKNOWLEDGEMENTS

Declared none.

REFERENCES

[1]   Gulick RM, Ribaudo HJ, Shikuma CM, *et al*. Triple-nucleoside regimens *versus* efavirenz-containing regimens for the initial treatment of HIV-1 infection. New Engl J Med 2004; 350(18): 1850-61.
[2]   Riddler SA, Haubrich R, DiRienzo AG, *et al*. Class-sparing regimens for initial treatment of HIV-1 infection. New Engl J Med 2008; 358(20): 2095-106.
[3]   NIH. Guidelines for the Use of Antiretroviral Agents in HIV-1-Infected Adults and Adolescents 2014 [cited 2014 June 29]. Available from:http: //aidsinfo.nih.gov/guidelines/html/1/adult-and-adolescent-arv-guidelines/0/.
[4]   Williams I, Churchill D, Anderson J, *et al*. British HIV Association guidelines for the treatment of HIV-1-positive adults with antiretroviral therapy 2012 (Updated November 2013. All changed text is cast in yellow highlight.). HIV Med 2014; 15 Suppl 1: 1-85.
[5]   IAS-USA. Antiretroviral Treatment of Adult HIV Infection 2012 [cited 2014 June 29]. Available from: http: //iasusa.org/content/antiretroviral-treatment-adult-hiv-infection-0.
[6]   EACS. EACS Guidelines 2014 [updated June 2014; cited 2014 June 29]. Available from: http: //www.eacsociety.org/Guidelines.aspx.
[7]   WHO. Antiretroviral therapy for HIV infection in adults and adolescents: recommendations for a public health approach 2010 [cited 2014 January 27]. Available from: *whqlibdoc.who.int/publications/2010/9789241599764_eng.pdf.*
[8]   WHO. Consolidated Guidelines on the Use of Antiretroviral Drugs for Treating and Preventing HIV Infection: Recommendations for a Public Health Approach 2013 [cited 2014 January 18]. Available from: *www.who.int/iris/bitstream/10665/85321/1/9789241505727_eng.pdf.*
[9]   Barré-Sinoussi F, Chermann JC, Rey F, *et al*. Isolation of a T-Lymphotropic Retrovirus from a Patient at Risk for Acquired Immune Deficiency Syndrome (AIDS). Science 1983; 220(4599): 868-71.
[10]   Gallo RC, Sarin PS, Gelmann EP, *et al*. Isolation of Human T-Cell Leukemia Virus in Acquired Immune Deficiency Syndrome (AIDS). Science 1983; 220(4599): 865-7.
[11]   Squires KE. An introduction to nucleoside and nucleotide analogues. Antivir Ther 2001; 6 Suppl 3: 1-14.
[12]   Wright K. AIDS therapy: First tentative signs of therapeutic promise. Nature 1986; 323(6086): 283-.
[13]   Wang LH, Begley J, St Claire RL, 3rd, *et al*. Pharmacokinetic and pharmacodynamic characteristics of emtricitabine support its once daily dosing for the treatment of HIV infection. AIDS Res Hum Retroviruses 2004; 20(11): 1173-82.

[14]   Wang LH, Wiznia AA, Rathore MH, *et al.* Pharmacokinetics and safety of single oral doses of emtricitabine in human immunodeficiency virus-infected children. Antimicrob Agents Chemother 2004; 48(1): 183-91.

[15]   Nakatani-Freshwater T, Taft DR. Renal excretion of emtricitabine I: effects of organic anion, organic cation, and nucleoside transport inhibitors on emtricitabine excretion. J Pharm Sci 2008; 97(12): 5401-10.

[16]   Colbers AP, Hawkins DA, Gingelmaier A, *et al.* The pharmacokinetics, safety and efficacy of tenofovir and emtricitabine in HIV-1-infected pregnant women. Aids 2013; 27(5): 739-48.

[17]   Ma Q, Okusanya OO, Smith PF, *et al.* Pharmacokinetic drug interactions with non-nucleoside reverse transcriptase inhibitors. Expert Opin Drug Metab Toxicol 2005; 1(3): 473-85.

[18]   Rathbun RC, Liedtke MD. Antiretroviral drug interactions: overview of interactions involving new and investigational agents and the role of therapeutic drug monitoring for management. Pharmaceutics 2011; 3(4): 745-81.

[19]   Drake SM. NNRTIs—a new class of drugs for HIV. J Antimicrob Chemother 2000; 45(4): 417-20.

[20]   Smith PF, DiCenzo R, Morse GD. Clinical pharmacokinetics of non-nucleoside reverse transcriptase inhibitors. Clin Pharmacokinet 2001; 40(12): 893-905.

[21]   Efavirenz: Non-nucleoside Reverse Transcriptase Inhibitors [Internet]. 2015. Available from: http: //aidsinfo.nih.gov/drugs/269/sustiva/0/professional.

[22]   Actavis. Arrow - Efavirenz: Efavirenz Tablets 600 mg. Actavis New Zealand Limited, Mt. Eden Central Business Park, 33a Normanby Road, Mt. Eden Auckland, New Zealand.2013 [updated 30 July 2013; cited 2015 March 30]. Available from: www.medsafe.govt.nz/Profs/Datasheet/a/arrowefavirenztab.pdf.

[23]   Chiappetta DA, Hocht C, Taira C, *et al.* Efavirenz-loaded polymeric micelles for pediatric anti-HIV pharmacotherapy with significantly higher oral bioavailability [corrected]. Nanomedicine (Lond) 2010; 5(1): 11-23.

[24]   Mukonzo JK, Nanzigu S, Rekic D, *et al.* HIV/AIDS patients display lower relative bioavailability of efavirenz than healthy subjects. Clin Pharmacokinet 2011; 50(8): 531-40.

[25]   Gaur PK, Mishra S, Bajpai M, *et al.* Enhanced oral bioavailability of efavirenz by solid lipid nanoparticles: *in vitro* drug release and pharmacokinetics studies. Biomed Res Int 2014; 2014: 363404.

[26]   Tshweu L, Katata L, Kalombo L, *et al.* Enhanced oral bioavailability of the antiretroviral efavirenz encapsulated in poly (epsilon-caprolactone) nanoparticles by a spray-drying method. Nanomedicine (Lond) 2014; 9(12): 1821-33.

[27]   Nanzigu S, Eriksen J, Makumbi F, *et al.* Pharmacokinetics of the nonnucleoside reverse transcriptase inhibitor efavirenz among HIV-infected Ugandans. HIV Med 2012; 13(4): 193-201.

[28]   Arab-Alameddine M, Di Iulio J, Buclin T, *et al.* Pharmacogenetics-based population pharmacokinetic analysis of efavirenz in HIV-1-infected individuals. Clin Pharmacol Ther 2009; 85(5): 485-94.

[29]   Ward BA, Gorski JC, Jones DR, *et al.* The cytochrome P450 2B6 (CYP2B6) is the main catalyst of efavirenz primary and secondary metabolism: implication for HIV/AIDS therapy and utility of efavirenz as a substrate marker of CYP2B6 catalytic activity. J Pharmacol Exp Ther 2003; 306(1): 287-300.

[30]   Court M, Almutairi F, Greenblatt DJ, *et al.* Identification of Isoniazid as a Potent Inhibitor of CYP2A6-mediated Efavirenz 7-hydroxylation in CYP2B6*6 Genotyped human Liver Microsomes. Conference on Retrovirus and Opportunistic Infections; March 3-6th 2013; Georgia World Conference Centre: CROI; 2013.

[31]   Wen X, Wang JS, Neuvonen PJ, *et al.* Isoniazid is a mechanism-based inhibitor of cytochrome P450 1A2, 2A6, 2C19 and 3A4 isoforms in human liver microsomes. Eur J Clin Pharmacol 2002; 57(11): 799-804.

[32]   Belanger AS, Caron P, Harvey M, *et al.* Glucuronidation of the antiretroviral drug efavirenz by UGT2B7 and an *in vitro* investigation of drug-drug interaction with zidovudine. Drug Metab Dispos 2009; 37(9): 1793-6.

[33]   Colic A, Alessandrini M, Pepper MS. Pharmacogenetics of CYP2B6, CYP2A6 and UGT2B7 in HIV treatment in African populations: focus on efavirenz and nevirapine. Drug Metab Rev 2014: 1-13.

[34]   Habtewold A, Amogne W, Makonnen E, *et al*. Long-term effect of efavirenz autoinduction on plasma/peripheral blood mononuclear cell drug exposure and CD4 count is influenced by UGT2B7 and CYP2B6 genotypes among HIV patients. J Antimicrob Chemother 2011.

[35]   Kwara A, Lartey M, Sagoe KW, *et al*. CYP2B6, CYP2A6 and UGT2B7 genetic polymorphisms are predictors of efavirenz mid-dose concentration in HIV-infected patients. AIDS 2009; 23(16): 2101-6.

[36]   Habtewold A, Amogne W, Makonnen E, *et al*. Pharmacogenetic and pharmacokinetic aspects of CYP3A induction by efavirenz in HIV patients. Pharmacogenomics J 2013; 13(6): 484-9.

[37]   Kappelhoff BS, van Leth F, MacGregor TR, *et al*. Nevirapine and efavirenz pharmacokinetics and covariate analysis in the 2NN study. Antivir Ther 2005; 10(1): 145-55.

[38]   Michaud V, Kreutz Y, Skaar T, *et al*. Efavirenz-mediated induction of omeprazole metabolism is CYP2C19 genotype dependent. Pharmacogenomics J 2013.

[39]   Nanzigu S. Host Variabilities Influencing HIV/ART Outcomes Scholars' Press; 2013. Available from: http: //www.amazon.com/Host-Variabilities-Influencing-Outcomes-Pharmacokinetics/dp/3639702190.

[40]   Ngaimisi E, Mugusi S, Minzi OM, *et al*. Long-term efavirenz autoinduction and its effect on plasma exposure in HIV patients. Clin Pharmacol Ther 2010; 88(5): 676-84.

[41]   Yimer G, Amogne W, Habtewold A, *et al*. High plasma efavirenz level and CYP2B6*6 are associated with efavirenz-based HAART-induced liver injury in the treatment of naive HIV patients from Ethiopia: a prospective cohort study. Pharmacogenomics J 2012; 12(6): 499-506.

[42]   Zhu M, Kaul S, Nandy P, *et al*. Model-Based Approach To Characterize Efavirenz Autoinduction and Concurrent Enzyme Induction with Carbamazepine. Antimicrob Agents Chemother 2009; 53(6): 2346-53.

[43]   Faucette SR, Zhang TC, Moore R, *et al*. Relative activation of human pregnane X receptor *versus* constitutive androstane receptor defines distinct classes of CYP2B6 and CYP3A4 inducers. Journal of Pharmacol Exp Ther. 2007; 320(1): 72-80.

[44]   Robertson SM, Maldarelli F, Natarajan V, *et al*. Efavirenz induces CYP2B6-mediated hydroxylation of bupropion in healthy subjects. J Acquir Immune Defic Syndr 2008; 49(5): 513-9.

[45]   Hariparsad N, Nallani SC, Sane RS, *et al*. Induction of CYP3A4 by efavirenz in primary human hepatocytes: comparison with rifampin and phenobarbital. J Clin Pharmacol 2004; 44(11): 1273-81.

[46]   Haas DW, Gebretsadik T, Mayo G, *et al*. Associations between CYP2B6 polymorphisms and pharmacokinetics after a single dose of nevirapine or efavirenz in African americans. J Infect Dis 2009; 199(6): 872-80.

[47]   Rotger M, Tegude H, Colombo S, *et al*. Predictive value of known and novel alleles of CYP2B6 for efavirenz plasma concentrations in HIV-infected individuals. Clin Pharmacol Ther 2007; 81(4): 557-66.

[48]   Burger D, van der Heiden I, la Porte C, *et al*. Interpatient variability in the pharmacokinetics of the HIV non-nucleoside reverse transcriptase inhibitor efavirenz: the effect of gender, race, and CYP2B6 polymorphism. Br J Clin Pharmacol 2006; 61(2): 148-54.

[49]   Ribaudo HJ, Haas DW, Tierney C, *et al*. Pharmacogenetics of plasma efavirenz exposure after treatment discontinuation: an Adult AIDS Clinical Trials Group Study. Clin Infect Dis 2006; 42(3): 401-7.

[50]   Mukonzo JK, Roshammar D, Waako P, *et al*. A novel polymorphism in ABCB1 gene, CYP2B6*6 and sex predict single-dose efavirenz population pharmacokinetics in Ugandans. Br J Clin Pharmacol 2009; 68(5): 690-9.

[51]   Nyakutira C, Roshammar D, Chigutsa E, *et al*. High prevalence of the CYP2B6 516G-->T(*6) variant and effect on the population pharmacokinetics of efavirenz in HIV/AIDS outpatients in Zimbabwe. Eur J Clin Pharmacol 2008; 64(4): 357-65.

[52]   Mukonzo JK, Owen JS, Ogwal-Okeng J, *et al*. Pharmacogenetic-based efavirenz dose modification: suggestions for an African population and the different CYP2B6 genotypes. PLoS One 2014; 9(1): e86919.

[53]   von Moltke LL, Greenblatt DJ, Granda BW, *et al*. Inhibition of Human Cytochrome P450 Isoforms by Nonnucleoside Reverse Transcriptase Inhibitors. J Clin Pharmacol 2001; 41(1): 85-91.

[54]   Weiss J, Herzog M, Konig S, *et al*. Induction of multiple drug transporters by efavirenz. J Pharmacol Sci 2009; 109(2): 242-50.

[55]   Dona C, Soriano V, Barreiro P, *et al*. [Toxicity associated to efavirenz in HIV-infected persons enrolled in an expanded access program]. Med Clin (Barc) 2000; 115(9): 337-8.

[56]   Munoz-Moreno JA, Fumaz CR, Ferrer MJ, *et al*. Neuropsychiatric symptoms associated with efavirenz: prevalence, correlates, and management. A neurobehavioral review. AIDS Rev 2009; 11(2): 103-9.

[57]   Rotger M, Colombo S, Furrer H, *et al*. Influence of CYP2B6 polymorphism on plasma and intracellular concentrations and toxicity of efavirenz and nevirapine in HIV-infected patients. Pharmacogenet Genomics 2005; 15(1): 1-5.

[58]   Usami O, Ashino Y, Komaki Y, *et al*. Efavirenz-induced neurological symptoms in rare homozygote CYP2B6 *2/*2 (C64T). Int J STD AIDS 2007; 18(8): 575-6.

[59]   Nijhawan AE, Zachary KC, Kwara A, *et al*. Status epilepticus resulting from severe efavirenz toxicity in an HIV-infected patient. AIDS Read 2008; 18(7): 386-8, C3.

[60]   Mollan KR, Smurzynski M, Eron JJ, *et al*. Association between efavirenz as initial therapy for HIV-1 infection and increased risk for suicidal ideation or attempted or completed suicide: an analysis of trial data. Ann Intern Med 2014; 161(1): 1-10.

[61]   Ena J, Amador C, Benito C, *et al*. Risk and determinants of developing severe liver toxicity during therapy with nevirapine-and efavirenz-containing regimens in HIV-infected patients. Int J STD AIDS 2003; 14(11): 776-81.

[62]   HIV Drug Resistance Database: NNRTI Resistance Notes [Internet]. 2014 [cited 2015, March 30]. Available from: http: //hivdb.stanford.edu/DR/NNRTIResiNote.html.

[63]   Alcaro S, Alteri C, Artese A, *et al*. Docking analysis and resistance evaluation of clinically relevant mutations associated with the HIV-1 non-nucleoside reverse transcriptase inhibitors nevirapine, efavirenz and etravirine. ChemMedChem 2011; 6(12): 2203-13.

[64]   Gallien S, Charreau I, Nere ML, *et al*. Archived HIV-1 DNA resistance mutations to rilpivirine and etravirine in successfully treated HIV-1-infected individuals pre-exposed to efavirenz or nevirapine. J Antimicrob Chemother 2015; 70(2): 562-5.

[65]   James C, Preininger L, Sweet M. Rilpivirine: a second-generation nonnucleoside reverse transcriptase inhibitor. Am J Health Syst Pharm 2012; 69(10): 857-61.

[66]   Efavirenz: Resistance   [Internet].   2015.   Available   from: http: //www.aidsmap.com/Resistance/page/1730988/#ref1525231.

[67]   Koval CE, Dykes C, Wang J, *et al*. Relative replication fitness of efavirenz-resistant mutants of HIV-1: correlation with frequency during clinical therapy and evidence of compensation for the reduced fitness of K103N + L100I by the nucleoside resistance mutation L74V. Virology 2006; 353(1): 184-92.

[68]   Ait-Khaled M, Rakik A, Griffin P, *et al*. HIV-1 reverse transcriptase and protease resistance mutations selected during 16-72 weeks of therapy in isolates from antiretroviral therapy-experienced patients receiving abacavir/efavirenz/amprenavir in the CNA2007 study. Antivir Ther 2003; 8(2): 111-20.

[69]   Chin BS, Shin HS, Kim G, *et al*. Increase of HIV-1 K103N Transmitted Drug Resistance and Its Association with Efavirenz Use in South Korea. AIDS Res Hum Retroviruses 2015.

[70]   Crawford KW, Njeru D, Maswai J, *et al*. Occurrence of etravirine/rilpivirine-specific resistance mutations selected by efavirenz and nevirapine in Kenyan patients with non-B HIV-1 subtypes failing antiretroviral therapy. AIDS 2014; 28(3): 442-5.

[71]   Cohen CJ, Andrade-Villanueva J, Clotet B, *et al*. Rilpivirine *versus* efavirenz with two background nucleoside or nucleotide reverse transcriptase inhibitors in treatment-naive adults infected with HIV-1 (THRIVE): a phase 3, randomised, non-inferiority trial. Lancet 2011; 378(9787): 229-37.

[72]   FDA. Edurant (Rilpivirine): Highlights of Prescribing information 2011 [cited 2014 June 29]. Available from: http: //www.accessdata.fda.gov/drugsatfda_docs/label/2011/202022s000lbl.pdf.

[73]   Janssen. Intelence (etravirine) tablets for oral use: Full prescribing information 2008 [cited 2014 June 29]. Available from: *www.intelence.com/hcp/full-prescribing-information*.

[74]   DHHS. DHHS Panel on Antiretroviral Guidelines for Adults and Adolescents, "Guidelines for the Use of Antiretroviral Agents in HIV-1-Infected Adults and Adolescents, Department of Health and Human Services," February 12, 2013.

[75]   Gutierrez-Valencia A, Martin-Pena R, Torres-Cornejo A, *et al*. Intracellular and plasma pharmacokinetics of 400 mg of etravirine once daily *versus* 200 mg of etravirine twice daily in HIV-infected patients. J Antimicrob Chemother 2012; 67(3): 681-4.

[76]   Letendre S, Ellis RJ, Deutsch R, *et al*. Correlates of Time-to-Loss-of-Viral-Response in CSF and Plasma in the CHARTER Cohort: CPE Score predicts CSF suppression 2010 [cited 2014 June 29]. Available from: http: //www.natap.org/2010/CROI/croi_71.htm.

[77]   Scholler-Gyure M, Boffito M, Pozniak AL, *et al*. Effects of different meal compositions and fasted state on the oral bioavailability of etravirine. Pharmacotherapy 2008; 28(10): 1215-22.

[78]   Giguere P, la Porte C, Zhang G, *et al*. Pharmacokinetics of darunavir, etravirine and raltegravir in an HIV-infected patient on haemodialysis. Aids 2009. p. 740-2.

[79]   Kakuda T, Green B, Morrish G, *et al*. Population pharmacokinetics of etravirine in HIV-1-infected treatment-experienced children and adolescents (6-17 years): week 24 primary analysis of the phase II PIANO   trial   2011   [cited   2014   July   7].   Available   from: http: //pag.ias2011.org/abstracts.aspx?aid=4842.

[80]   Kakuda TN, Schöller-Gyüre M, Peeters M, *et al*., editors. Pharmacokinetics of etravirine (ETR; TMC125) are not affected by sex, age, race, use of enfuvirtide (ENF) or treatment duration in HIV-1-infected subjects.

[81]   DHHS. DHHS Panel on Treatment of HIV-Infected Pregnant Women and Prevention of Perinatal Transmission, "Recommendations for Use of Antiretroviral Drugs in Pregnant HIV-1-Infected Women for Maternal Health and Interventions to Reduce Perinatal HIV Transmission in the United States", March 28, 2014.

[82]   Izurieta P *et al*. Safety and pharmacokinetics of etravirine in pregnant HIV-infected women [abstract PE 4.1/6]. 12th European AIDS Conference, Cologne, November 11-14, 2009.

[83]   Nelson M, Stellbrink H-J, Podzamczer D, *et al*. A comparison of neuropsychiatric adverse events during 12 weeks of treatment with etravirine and efavirenz in a treatment-naive, HIV-1-infected population. Aids 2011; 25(3): 335-40.

[84]   Vingerhoets J, Tambuyzer L, Azijn H, *et al*. Resistance profile of etravirine: combined analysis of baseline genotypic and phenotypic data from the randomized, controlled Phase III clinical studies. Aids 2010; 24(4): 503-14.

APPENDIX 1

Table 5. Key pharmacokinetic parameters for selected reverse transcriptase inhibitors [11, 21]

Generic name	Dosage form (s)	Route (s) used	Bioavailability after oral route (%)	Volume of Distribution (L/kg)	Protein Binding (%)	Metabolism/ elimination	Half-life (H)	Effect of CYP450 Induces	Effect of CYP450 Inhibits	Drug interactions
Emtricitabine	200mg mg (adults) OD or 6mg/kg	Oral	93% (capsule) 75%(oral solution)	1.4	<4	Renal elimination, Limited oxidation and conjugation	10	Limited data	MRP1 MRP2 MRP3	Trimethoprim reduces renal secretion by 60%
Zidovudine	300mg	Oral Parenteral	64%	1.6	25 -38	Hepatic glucuronidation	1 (0.5-2.9)	None	None	Intra-class competition for phosphorylation Drugs interfering with phase II conjugation
Abacavir	300mg BD or 600mg OD	Oral	83% (65-107).	0.86	50	alcohol dehydrogenase and glucuronidation	2	None at clinical relevance	None at clinical relevance	ethanol causes the AUC of abacavir
Lamivudine GlaxoSmithKline	300mg	Oral	86	1.3	<36	Renal elimination Minor hepatic sulfation	5-7	None	None	Competition for intracellular phosphorylation with Zalcitabine
Tenofovir	300mg OD	Oral Injectable	25% but increased by 40% if taken with a fatty meal	1.2-1.3	<7	Intracellular hydrolysis	17 (12-18) (plasma) 150 (intracellular)	CYP2C9	CYP2E1	PIs inhibit intestinal Pgp causing dose-dependent increase in tenofovir
Efavirenz	600mg OD for adults	Oral	45%	40-55	>99	CYP2B6, 3A4, 1A2,	40-55	Extensive CYP450 Induction	Limited data	Multiple drug interactions- Rifampicin, ketoconazole,

CHAPTER 4

Integrase Inhibitors

Sarah Nanzigu[1,*] and Francis Xavier Kasujja[2]

[1]Department of Pharmacology and Therapeutics, Makerere University College of Health Science, Kampala-Uganda and [2]Médecins Sans Frontières, Harare, Zimbabwe

Abstract: Antiretroviral agents target specific steps in the HIV replication cycle. This chapter focuses on HIV DNA integration, a step catalyzed by the integrase enzyme. Appreciating the structure of this enzyme and its mechanism of action is vital to understanding how the drugs inhibit this step. The integrase enzyme constitutes vital domains and amino acids that can be drug targets during 3' processing (3'-P) and strand transfer (ST). Active against these processes are some derivatives of **Diketo Acids** (DKA), **Strylquinolones** (SQL) and **Phenyldipyrimidine (PDP)**. To date, three drugs active against strand transfer – Raltegravir, Elvitegravir and Dolutegravir – have been approved by the Food and Drug Authority (FDA). Several other agents are still undergoing pre-clinical and clinical trials. Integrase inhibitors are effective against HIV1 and HIV2, including multidrug resistant strains of HIV1. Therefore antiretroviral combinations containing these drugs are effective as first or second line regimens. Resistance to integrase inhibitors mainly follows amino acid substitutions in the catalytic core domain of the enzyme. Y143C/R, Q148H/K/R and N155H mutations have been attributed to Raltegravir and Elvitegravir resistance. These mutations, however, have minimal effect on the action of Dolutegravir.

Keywords: Integrase Inhibitors, Antiretroviral Drugs, HIV, Raltegravir, Elvitegravir, Dolutegravir, Integrase, Diketo acids, Strand transfer inhibitors, INSTI.

INTRODUCTION

Integration – the incorporation of the double stranded viral DNA (dsDNA) formed during reverse transcription, into host DNA [1] – involves six steps [2]:

1. Binding of integrase enzyme to viral DNA,

2. Processing of the HIV 3-prime ends – also called 3' processing (3'-P),

3. Nuclear Translocation of the DNA-integrase pre-integration complex,

*Corresponding author Sarah Nanzigu: Department of Pharmacology and Therapeutics, Makerere University College of Health Sciences, Kampala, Uganda; Tel: 25678484304, Fax: 256414532947;
E-mails: snanzigu@yahoo.com; snanzigu@chs.mak.ac.ug

Gene D. Morse and Sarah Nanzigu (Eds)

4. Binding of the pre-integration complex to host DNA,

5. Transfer of viral DNA into host DNA – also called strand transfer (ST) and,

6. Repair of the gaps formed during ST – also called gap repair.

All the drugs registered to date that target integration, act against the strand transfer process. In this chapter, however, both 3' processing (step 2) and strand transfer (step 5), the two processes catalyzed by the integrase enzyme [1, 3-5], are discussed.

THE INTEGRASE ENZYME

The Structure of the Integrase Enzyme

The integrase enzyme belongs to the family of polynucleotidyl transferases [6], and it comprises of three distinct domains: the **C-Terminal Domain (CTD),** the **N-Terminal Domain (NTD)** and the **Catalytic Core Domain (CCD)**[6, 7]. The presence of all three domains is vital for integration. The CCD contains the enzyme active site while the NTD and CTD are active during 3' processing and strand-transfer. Alone, the CCD catalyzes a reverse disintegration reaction [7].

To activate the enzyme, a trio of amino acids contained in the CCD – D64, D116 and E152 – coordinates the binding of CCD with a divalent metal such as magnesium (Mg^{2+}) or manganese (Mn^{2+})[7]. D64 and D116 form a coordination complex with the metal; D116 and E152 also possibly form another metal coordination-complex after the binding of HIV integrase to the dsDNA substrate (Fig. **1**). The bound metals are thought to coordinate the bonding of the enzyme with viral DNA during 3'-P and ST [7]. Drug action and resistance selection are highly dependent on the amino acid trio and the bound metals [8, 9]

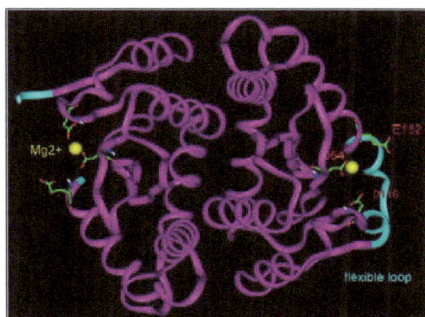

http://www.msg.ucsf.edu/stroud/structure/hiv_int.htm

Fig. (1). The Catalytic Core Domain (CCD) of the Integrase enzyme: The amino acids D64, D116 and E152 coordinate binding of divalent metals in order to activate the domain.

Integrase Enzyme Activity

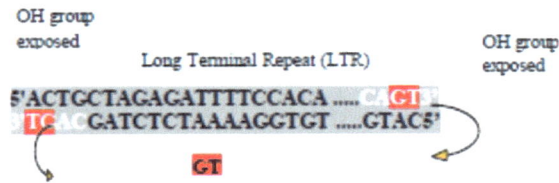

Fig. (2). The long terminal repeat sequence of the HIV dsDNA. The integrase enzyme cleaves off the GT dinucleotide at the 3' ends of viral DNA in preparation for insertion into the host DNA [2, 6, 10].

In preparation for viral DNA integration into host DNA, integrase cleaves the 3' end of viral DNA, removing the GT dinucleotide [6] and exposing an intermediate reactive hydroxyl group of the CA dinucleotides at the 3' end (3'-hydroxy group). The action concurrently creates a dinucleotide overhang at the 5' end (Fig. **2**).

In the subsequent step, retroviral integrase catalyzes strand transfer. Viral DNA is inserted into a selected region of the host cell DNA (Fig. **4**); specifically, the enzyme catalyzes the initial reaction in which the 3'-hydroxy group of HIV DNA attacks host DNA. This separates the host DNA base pair bonds located between the cut ends of the viral DNA, paving way for the joining of the 3'-hydroxyl groups of the viral DNA with the 5'-phosphate ends of host DNA.

The insertion of the new viral DNA and the presence of DNA gaps in unpaired regions induce a host cellular DNA damage repair response: gap repair [2, 11]. The fully-integrated DNA is at this stage called the provirus.

INTEGRASE INHIBITORS

In principle, the drugs or compounds that are active against integration may target any of the above 6 steps. However, all the currently known integrase inhibitors (Table **1**) specifically block the two processes catalyzed by the integrase enzyme, namely, 3' processing and strand transfer.

Integrase inhibitors block the integration of viral dsDNA into the host cell's chromosomal DNA [19]. No mammalian homologue of the integrase enzyme exists, a fact that promotes the use of these agents. Most of the currently approved integrase inhibitors (Table **1**) are derivatives of Diketo acids (DKAs).

Mechanism of Action

Generally, DKA derivatives compete with the targeted substrate, HIV DNA, for viral integrase during strand transfer [8, 12, 13]. The DKA inhibition mechanism is metal dependent: the inhibitor interacts with the divalent metal at the CCD site, and the diketo group plays a role in metal chelation [8, 9] (Fig. **3**).

Table 1. Chemical compounds and drugs that inhibit integrase

Chemical group	Targeted Step	Lead compounds	Resultant Drugs
Diketo acid derivatives (DKA) [7, 12-14]	**Strand transfer:** The compounds compete with HIV DNA substrate for the integrase enzyme. Some of the compounds chelate the Mg^{2+}/Mn^{2+} metals in the CCD domain	L-731988 L-708906 L-870812 L-870 810 S-1360 5CITEP	L708906 to Raltegravir [15, 16] and Elvitegravir
Strylquinolone derivatives (SQL) [7, 17]	**Mainly 3' processing, and Strand Transfer to a lesser extent:** The compounds compete with the HIV DNA substrate for integrase. Some may chelate the divalent Mg^{2+}/Mn^{2+} metals in the CCD	FZ41 KHD161	Research ongoing
Phenyldipyrimidines (PDPs) [7, 18]	**Mainly Strand transfer, and 3' processing to some extent**: Some of these compounds have activity against Reverse Transcriptase	V-165	Research ongoing

DKAs can inhibit strand transfer at much lower concentrations compared to those required to inhibit 3' processing (about 30-70 folds) [12]. Although the structure-activity relationship of the integrase is distinct, similarities with the reverse nuclease exist; therefore, DKAs may inhibit RNase at very high concentrations [12].

Development of Resistance

Resistance to current integrase inhibitors usually follows mutations in the sequences of the three amino acids (D64, D116 or E152) that coordinate the binding of the divalent metal in the catalytic core domain (CCD) of the integrase enzyme.

RALTEGRAVIR

Background

Raltegravir is a first generation integrase inhibitor that was approved by FDA in 2007. It is a derivative of the DKA, L-708906 (Fig. **3**) [13, 15].

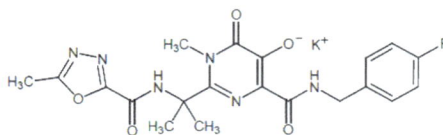

Fig. (3). Chemical structure of Raltegravir ($C_{20}H_{20}FKN_6O_5$), molecular weight 482.51g/mol. The K^+ is involved in chelating divalent metals [13, 15, 20]

Mechanism of Action

Raltegravir competitively inhibits the strand transfer activity of integrase. It is also believed to chelate the divalent metal ion at the CCD.

INTEGRASE INHIBITOR (RALTEGRAVIR)

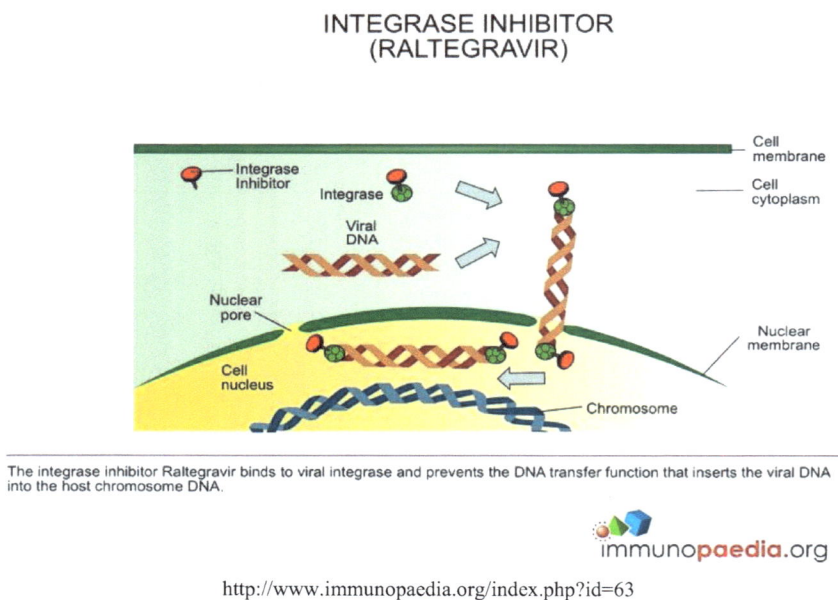

The integrase inhibitor Raltegravir binds to viral integrase and prevents the DNA transfer function that inserts the viral DNA into the host chromosome DNA.

immuno**paedia**.org

http://www.immunopaedia.org/index.php?id=63

Fig. (4). Illustration of the mechanism of action of Integrase Inhibitor Raltegravir.

Dosing Information

Dosage forms of Raltegravir include three tablet forms: the 400mg is film-coated, the 100mg is chewable, and so is the 25mg preparation. Chewable tablets give better bioavailability compared to those that are film coated. The dosing of this drug for both adults and children [21] is as follows:

- For adults 400mg twice a day is recommended, administered in combination with other antiretroviral agents,

- Children older than or 12 years of age may take 400mg twice daily,

- Children, 6-12 years and ≥25kg receive 400 mg film-coated tablets twice daily or weight based chewable tablets up to 300mg twice daily,

- Children 2-6 years and ≥10kg receive weight based chewable tablets, up to 300 mg.

- The weight based dose is 6mg/kg/twice daily [20, 21].

Drug safety for children less than 2 years has not been established.

Pharmacokinetics of Raltegravir

The bioavailability of an oral 400mg dose is estimated to be 30%, and the time to maximum concentration is 3 hours (T_{max}=3 hrs) [22]. The drug reaches steady state concentrations in 2 days with an average maximum concentration (C_{max}) of 4.5µmol/L[23] and a mean area under the curve over 12 hours (AUC0-12hr) of 14.2 µmol/L*hr. The concentration at 12 hours after an oral dose (C_{12}) is 142 nM [21, 23].

A fat diet and high pH increase drug absorption; a high fatty meal causes a 2-fold increase in AUC and C_{max}, and a 4-fold increase in C_{12}. Raltegravir is 83% plasma protein bound [21]. The drug exhibits a high inter-patient (>200-fold) and intra-patient variability (>100fold) in C_{12} post-dose concentrations [24]. Earlier studies showed that the AUC and C_{max} increased when the dose was raised from 100mg to 1600mg; at 1600mg, the C_{max} was 4 times higher than the value at 400mg [21].

Drug elimination is biphasic. The mean alpha phase is 1 hour while the beta phase is 9 hours (range 7-12hours) [16, 23].

Pharmacogenetics of Raltegravir

Raltegravir undergoes glucuronidation in human hepatic microsomes. The glucuronidation of raltegravir is mainly catalyzed by UGT1A1, with minor contributions from UGT1A9 and UGT1A3. RAL is also a substrate of P-glycoprotein (P-gp). A small proportion of the drug is excreted unchanged in urine.

Although UGT1A1*28/*28 is reported to reduce the metabolism of raltegravir giving a C_{12} which is about 2-fold higher than the wild type (UGT1A1*1/*1), no dosage adjustments are required [21, 25]. A 2-fold increase in the AUC of

Raltegravir and a reduction in the minimum concentration (C_{min}) of up to 68% may have no clinical relevance. No gender or racial differences in the pharmacogenomics of the drug have, so far, been reported.

Drug Interactions

Rifampicin may reduce the AUC of Raltegravir by 40%, and plasma concentrations may reduce by 61% following UGT1A1 induction. Raltegravir dosage adjustment to 800mg twice daily for patients on rifampicin has been suggested [22, 23].

Raltegravir has not been shown to inhibit or induce the CYP group of enzymes nor the P-glycoprotein or UGT group. However, Atazanavir, a retroviral protease inhibitor, increases Raltegravir plasma levels through the inhibition of UGT1A1[23] while Tenofovir and Ritonavir-boosted Taprinavir may reduce its plasma concentration by 64% and 55% respectively. Similarly, antacids containing divalent metal ions when administered within 2 hours of Raltegravir may chelate the drug, interfering with its absorption and resulting in a 67% reduction of the C_{12} [21, 24]. So far, all these effects are not thought to be of clinical relevance [21, 23, 24].

Therapeutic Uses

Raltegravir is active against HIV 1 and HIV 2 including both CCR5-tropic and CXCR4-tropic strains, as well as multidrug resistant strains [26, 27]. The drug is thought to work additively or synergistically with both nucleoside and non-nucleoside reverse transcriptase inhibitors [28, 29]. Raltegravir-based combinations show durable viral suppression up to 5 years, including among patients with multidrug resistance HIV 1 strains [30]. The drug is shown to have a long term efficacy as measured by virological control and CD4 gain that was better than that seen in Efavirenz-based regimens, including in patients with high baseline viral load [23, 31].

Drug efficacy in HIV 1 non-B subtypes is similar to that seen in the B-subtype. Furthermore, the efficacy and safety in children aged 2-28 years is similar to that in adults [32].

Adverse Drug Reactions

Raltegravir-based combinations are better tolerated and have fewer adverse reactions compared to Efavirenz-based combinations [31]. However, minor side effects have been reported in about 2% of the patients including dizziness, headache, nausea, excessive tiredness and sleep disturbances [33]. Life threatening skin reactions, including Steven Johnson reactions and toxic epidermal necrolysis, may occur in less than 2% of the patients [20, 21].

Hepatic aminotransferases may be elevated up to grade-4 level, just like in the case for Efavirenz-based regimens [21]; however, gastrointestinal disorders may be more frequent in Raltegravir-based regimens [21], and immune reconstitution syndrome was observed during clinical trials. Raltegravir should be used with caution in patients at increased risk of myopathy or rhabdomyolysis [31].

Squamous cell carcinoma of the nasal pharynx was observed in female rats dosed with Raltegravir at 600 mg/kg/day for 104 weeks. This has not been observed in humans [20]. The drug crosses the placental barrier giving fetal placenta concentration of about 2% of the maternal plasma concentrations but no teratogenic effects were observed after pregnant rabbits and rats were administered with Raltegravir doses of up to 1000mg/kg/day [21]. At doses of 600mg/kg/day in breast feeding rats, the drug concentration was 3 times higher in breast milk as compared to that found in maternal plasma, but this was not associated with any adverse effects in the breastfed babies [20].

HIV Resistance to Raltegravir

Resistance to DKA derivatives is metal dependent [8] just like their mechanism of action. Mutations in any of the three amino acids that are adjacent to D64 and E152 have been found to confer resistance to Diketo acids [8]. Clinically important mutations include amino acid substitutions at various positions including 143 to C, H or R; or substitutions at positions 140, 148 or 155. Viral strains with the resultant mutations – Y143C/H/R, Q148H/K/R, and N155H – show reduced susceptibility to Raltegravir [34-36].

Occurrence of secondary mutations like E92Q in association with the N155H mutation, and/or G140S occurring in association with the Q148H mutation return integrase activity back to pre-treatment levels even in the presence of the drug [34-36]. Yet, a single G140S mutation has profound effect on strand transfer but little effect on 3' processing [36]. The G140S-Q148H double mutant can be cross-transmitted to Elvitegravir [36].

Other mutations identified as contributing to virological failure include T66A and L74I [34]. The G140S/Q148R, N155H and E92Q/N155H mutations also lead to

HIV2 resistance to Raltegravir [37, 38]. Other Raltegravir mutations detected in HIV 2 patients include T97A/N155H and T97A/Y143C. The G140S/Q148R and E92Q/N155H, T97A/N155H and T97A/Y143C double-mutations can persist for several months after the administration of Raltegravir has been stopped [38, 39]. In one study, the integrase genotypic pattern of one patient was seen to have evolved to T97A/Y143G eighteen months after Raltegravir had been stopped due to resistance [39].

ELVITEGRAVIR (GS-9137)

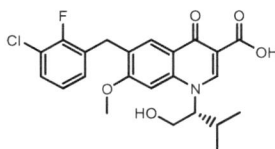

Fig. (5). Chemical structure of Elvitegravir ($C_{23}H_{23}ClFNO_5$), 447.883 g/mol [40-42].

Elvitegravir is a second generation integrase inhibitor approved by FDA in 2012. It is a monoketo acid resulting from early modification of the DKA motif (Fig. **5**), and hence retains some DKA functional groups [41-43]. These properties have a bearing on its mode of action and its selection of some of the resistance strains observed with Raltegravir.

Mechanism of Action

Like Raltegravir, Elvitegravir inhibits the integrase enzyme during strand transfer [44].

Pharmacokinetics and Pharmacogenetic Properties of Elvitegravir

The half-life ($T_{1/2}$) of unboosted Elvitegravir was shown to be 2-5 hours in animals; however, Ritonavir or Cobicistat-boosted Elvitegravir has a $T_{1/2}$ of 9hrs in humans [42]. For this reason, boosted Elvitegravir is administered once a day. The drug is primarily metabolized by the CYP3A4/5 group of enzymes, and later by UGT1A1/3[43].

Dosing

Stribild is a fixed dose drug combination containing Emtricitabine (200mg), Tenofovir disoproxil fumarate (300mg) and Cobicistat (150mg)-boosted Elvitegravir (150mg) (ELV/Cob+FTC+TDF [40]. The recommended dose is one tablet taken daily after a meal [40].

Therapeutic Uses

Elvitegravir has activity against HIV 2 and several HIV 1 isolates, namely, A, B, C, D, E, F G and O; it is also active against some strains that are resistant to NRTI, NNRTI, and PI [44].

Drug Interactions

Just like Raltegravir, the plasma concentration of Elvitegravir is reduced in the presence of the antituberculous drugs, Rifabutin and Rifampicin. Similarly, antacids administered within 2 hours of Elvitegravir reduce its plasma levels.

HIV Resistance to Elvitegravir

Resistance to Elvitegravir arises mainly from amino acid substitutions in the integrase CCD in a manner similar to the case of Raltegravir; however, the positions for the mutations might differ. The primary resistance mutations, T66I and E92Q, located in the CCD cause about 36-fold reduction in susceptibility to Elvitegravir while Q146P and S147G lead to 11-fold reduction in susceptibility. The secondary mutations – H51Y, Q95K, and E157Q – located proximal to these primary mutations confer a less than 10-fold reduction in susceptibility to Elvitegravir; however, multiple amino substitutions, including combinations of S147G with T66I/Q146P or E92Q, may cause a >300-fold reduction in susceptibility [44].

HIV-1 T66I/S153Y, a resistance strain selected by Raltegravir, results in high-level resistance to Elvitegravir. In addition, both L74M and S153Y mutations, in combination with T66I, are selected by other DKAs including Raltegravir.

DOLUTEGRAVIR S/GSK1349572

Dolutegravir is a second generation inhibitor of the strand integration process which was approved by the FDA in 2013. The drug has a molecular weight of 419.3821 g/mol.

Pharmacokinetics Properties and Therapeutic uses

Unboosted Dolutegravir has a long T1/2 of about 13-15 hours; it is therefore administered as a 50mg once daily dose in combination with other antiretroviral agents. Dolutegravir is mainly metabolized by the UGT1A1 while CYP3A4, UGT1A3, and UGT1A9 form minor metabolic pathways [45].

Dolutegravir is a substrate of the P-glycoprotein (P-gp) and the human breast cancer resistance protein (BCRP) but doesn't show any inhibitory or inductive effect on CYP450 enzymes [45].

Antiretroviral regimens containing Dolutegravir have so far shown better virological control at 48 weeks of therapy when compared to PI-based and Efavirenz-based regimens [46, 47]. The drug is non-inferior to Raltegravir as regards efficacy [43, 48]. Compared to other approved integrase inhibitors, Dolutegravir is less prone to resistance: it is efficacious among patients resistant to Raltegravir following Y143C/R, Q148H/K/R and N155H mutations [49, 50].

CONFLICT OF INTEREST

The authors confirm that this chapter contents have no conflict of interest.

ACKNOWLEDGEMENTS

Declared none.

REFERENCES

[1]   NIH. HIV Replication Cycle Steps in the HIV Replication Cycle 2012 [cited 21 Novmeber 2013]. Available from: http://www.niaid.nih.gov/topics/HIVAIDS/Understanding/Biology/pages/hiv-replicationcycle.aspx/
[2]   Craigie R. Genome-wide analysis of retroviral DNA integration. Nat Rev Microbiol 2005; 3:848-58.
[3]   Engelman A, Mizuuchi K,Craigie R. HIV-1 DNA integration: mechanism of viral DNA cleavage and DNA strand transfer. Cell 1991; 67(6): 1211-21.
[4]   Johnson AA, Santos W, Pais GC, *et al*. Integration requires a specific interaction of the donor DNA terminal 5'-cytosine with glutamine 148 of the HIV-1 integrase flexible loop. J Biol Chem 2006; 281(1): 461-7.
[5]   Johnson AA, Sayer JM, Yagi H, *et al*. Effect of DNA modifications on DNA processing by HIV-1 integrase and inhibitor binding: role of DNA backbone flexibility and an open catalytic site. J Biol Chem 2006; 281(43): 32428-38.
[6]   Guiot E, Carayon K, Delelis O, *et al*. Relationship between the Oligomeric Status of HIV-1 Integrase on DNA and Enzymatic Activity. J Biol Chem 2006; 281(32): 22707-19.
[7]   Pommier Y, Johnson AA,Marchand C. Integrase inhibitors to treat HIV/AIDS. Nat Rev Drug Discov 2005; 4(3): 236-48.
[8]   Grobler JA, Stillmock K, Hu B, *et al*. Diketo acid inhibitor mechanism and HIV-1 integrase: Implications for metal binding in the active site of phosphotransferase enzymes. Proceedings of the National Academy of Sciences 2002; 99(10): 6661-6.
[9]   Bacchi A, Carcelli M, Compari C, *et al*. Investigating the Role of Metal Chelation in HIV-1 Integrase Strand Transfer Inhibitors.   J Med Chem 2011; 54(24): 8407-20.
[10]   Panganiban AT, Temin HM. The retrovirus pol gene encodes a product required for DNA integration: identification of a retrovirus int locus. Proceedings of the National Academy of Sciences 1984; 81(24): 7885-9.
[11]   Craigie R. HIV Integrase, a Brief Overview from Chemistry to Therapeutics. J Biol Chem 2001; 276(26): 23213-6.

[12]   Espeseth AS, Felock P, Wolfe A, *et al*. HIV-1 integrase inhibitors that compete with the target DNA substrate define a unique strand transfer conformation for integrase. Proceedings of the National Academy of Sciences 2000; 97(21): 11244-9.

[13]   Hazuda DJ, Felock P, Witmer M, *et al*. Inhibitors of Strand Transfer That Prevent Integration and Inhibit HIV-1 Replication in Cells. Science 2000; 287(5453): 646-50.

[14]   Di Santo R, Costi R, Roux A, *et al*. Novel Bifunctional Quinolonyl Diketo Acid Derivatives as HIV-1 Integrase Inhibitors: Design, Synthesis, Biological Activities, and Mechanism of Action. J Med Chem 2006; 49(6): 1939-45.

[15]   Beare KD, Coster MJ, Rutledge PJ. Diketoacid inhibitors of HIV-1 integrase: from L-708,906 to raltegravir and beyond. Curr Med Chem 2012; 19(8): 1177-92.

[16]   Wiley. Modern Drug Synthesis. Hoboke, New Jersey: John Wiley & Sons; 2010. Available from: http://books.google.co.ug/books?id=NtdT5maa_pMC&pg=PP28&lpg=PP28&dq=Raltegravir,+DKA &source=bl&ots=0Ig73JAbBx&sig=0_bLGRGpuuSELvHdpn4Vh9- uzR0&hl=en&sa=X&ei=F6KXUvS9BJCMkAfxq4HgDQ&redir_esc=y#v=onepage&q=Raltegravir% 2C%20DKA&f=false/

[17]   Bonnenfant S, Thomas CM, Vita C, *et al*. Styrylquinolines, Integrase Inhibitors Acting Prior to Integration: a New Mechanism of Action for Anti-Integrase Agents. J Virol 2004; 78(11): 5728-36.

[18]   Pannecouque C, Pluymers W, B. VM, *et al*. New class of HIV integrase inhibitors that block viral replication in cell culture. Curr Biol 2002; 12(14): 1169-77.

[19]   Lataillade M, Kozal MJ. The hunt for HIV-1 integrase inhibitors. AIDS Patient Care STDS 2006; 20(7): 489-501.

[20]   Isentress® (Raltegravir). The Internet Drug Index 2013 [cited 03/12/2013]. Available from:http://www.rxlist.com/isentress-drug.htm.

[21]   Dohme MS. ISENTRESS® (raltegravir) film-coated tablets, for oral use. US Patent USA2013, 2007.

[22]   FDA. Centre for Drug Evaluation and Research: Application number 22-145. 2007.

[23]   Hicks C, Gulick RM. Raltegravir: The First HIV Type 1 Integrase Inhibitor. Clin Infect Dis 2009; 48(7): 931-9.

[24]   Kiser JJ, Bumpass JB, Meditz AL, *et al*. Effect of antacids on the pharmacokinetics of raltegravir in human immunodeficiency virus-seronegative volunteers. Antimicrob Agents Chemother 2010; 54(12): 4999-5003.

[25]   Wenning LA, Petry AS, Kost JT, *et al*. Pharmacokinetics of raltegravir in individuals with UGT1A1 polymorphisms. Clin Pharmacol Ther 2009; 85(6): 623-7.

[26]   Acton A. Integrases- Advances in Research and Application. 2013.

[27]   Grinsztejn B, Nguyen BY, Katlama C, *et al*. Safety and efficacy of the HIV-1 integrase inhibitor raltegravir (MK-0518) in treatment-experienced patients with multidrug-resistant virus: a phase II randomised controlled trial. Lancet 2007; 369(9569): 1261-9.

[28]   Charpentier C, Weiss L. Extended use of raltegravir in the treatment of HIV-1 infection: optimizing therapy. Infect Drug Resist 2010; 3: 103-14.

[29]   Okeke NL, Hicks C. Role of raltegravir in the management of HIV-1 infection. HIV/AIDS 2011; 3: 81-92.

[30]   Evering TH, Markowitz M. Raltegravir: an integrase inhibitor for HIV-1. Expert Opin Investig Drugs 2008; 17(3): 413-22.

[31]   Rockstroh JK, Lennox JL, DeJesus E, *et al*. Long-term Treatment With Raltegravir or Efavirenz Combined With Tenofovir/Emtricitabine for Treatment-Naive Human Immunodeficiency Virus-1– Infected Patients: 156-Week Results From STARTMRK. Clin Infect Dis 2011; 53(8): 807-16.

[32]   Nachman S, Acosta E, Zheng N, *et al*., editors. IMPAACT P1066: raltegravir (RAL) safety and efficacy in HIV infected (+) youth two to 18 years of age through week 48. 12th International AIDS Conference; July 22-27, 2012; Washington DC USA: AIDS.

[33]   Croxtall JD, Lyseng-Williamson KA, Perry CM. Raltegravir. Drugs 2008; 68(1): 131-8.

[34]   Charpentier C, Karmochkine M, Laureillard D, *et al*. Drug resistance profiles for the HIV integrase gene in patients failing raltegravir salvage therapy. HIV Med 2008; 9(9): 765-70.

[35]   Buck ML, Hofer KN, McCarthy MW, Cogut SB. Use of Raltegravir in Pediatric HIV-1 Infection. MedScape 2012.

[36]   Metifiot M, Maddali K, Naumova A, *et al*. Biochemical and pharmacological analyses of HIV-1 integrase flexible loop mutants resistant to raltegravir. Biochemistry 2010; 49(17): 3715-22.

[37]   Ni XJ, Delelis O, Charpentier C, *et al*. G140S/Q148R and N155H mutations render HIV-2 Integrase resistant to raltegravir whereas Y143C does not. Retrovirology 2011; 8: 68.

[38]   Charpentier C, Roquebert B, Delelis O, *et al*. Hot spots of integrase genotypic changes leading to HIV-2 resistance to raltegravir. Antimicrob Agents Chemother 2011; 55(3): 1293-5.

[39]   Charpentier C, Larrouy L, Matheron S, *et al*. Long-lasting persistence of integrase resistance mutations in HIV-2-infected patients after raltegravir withdrawal. Antiviral Ther 2011; 16(6): 937-40.

[40]   Gilead. Stibild Package Inser. FDA 2012.

[41]   Sato M, Motomura T, Aramaki H, *et al*. Novel HIV-1 Integrase Inhibitors Derived from Quinolone Antibiotics. J Med Chem 2006; 49(5): 1506-8.

[42]   Serrao E, Odde S, Ramkumar K, Neamati N. Raltegravir, elvitegravir, and metoogravir: the birth of "me-too" HIV-1 integrase inhibitors. Retrovirology 2009; 6(1): 25.

[43]   Quashie PK, Sloan RD, Wainberg MA. Novel therapeutic strategies targeting HIV integrase. BMC medicine 2012; 10: 34.

[44]   Shimura K, Kodama E, Sakagami Y, *et al*. Broad Antiretroviral Activity and Resistance Profile of the Novel Human Immunodeficiency Virus Integrase Inhibitor Elvitegravir (JTK-303/GS-9137). J Virol 2008; 82(2): 764-74.

[45]   Reese MJ, Savina PM, Generaux GT, *et al*. *In vitro* investigations into the roles of drug transporters and metabolizing enzymes in the disposition and drug interactions of dolutegravir, a HIV integrase inhibitor. Drug metabolism and disposition: the biological fate of chemicals 2013; 41(2): 353-61.

[46]   Feinberg J, Clotet B, Khuong MA, *et al*. H-1464a - Once-Daily Dolutegravir (DTG) is Superior to Darunavir/Ritonavir (DRV/r) in Antiretroviral-Naive Adults: 48 Week Results from FLAMINGO (ING114915) In: Mascolin, editor. 53rd ICAAC; Thursday, Sep 12, 2013, 3:00 PM - 5:30 PM Denver, Co2013.

[47]   Mascolin M, editor Integrase Inhibitor Dolutegravir First ARV Superior to Efavirenz in ART-Naive. 52nd ICAAC; September 9-12, 2012; San Francisco.

[48]   Raffi F, Rachlis A, Stellbrink HJ, *et al*. Once-daily dolutegravir *versus* raltegravir in antiretroviral-naive adults with HIV-1 infection: 48 week results from the randomised, double-blind, non-inferiority SPRING-2 study. Lancet 2013; 381(9868): 735-43.

[49]   Vavro C, Hasan S, Madsen H, *et al*. Prevalent polymorphisms in wild-type HIV-1 integrase are unlikely to engender drug resistance to dolutegravir (S/GSK1349572). Antimicrob Agents Chemother 2013; 57(3): 1379-84.

[50]   DeAnda F, Hightower KE, Nolte RT, *et al*. Dolutegravir Interactions with HIV-1 Integrase-DNA: Structural Rationale for Drug Resistance and Dissociation Kinetics. PloS one 2013; 8(10).

Protease Enzyme Inhibition

Rebecca A. Sumner[1,2,3], Cindy J. Bednasz[1,2], Qing Ma[1,2] and Gene D. Morse[1,2,*]

[1]*Translational Pharmacology Research Core, New York State Center of Excellence in Bioinformatics and Life Sciences, USA;* [2]*School of Pharmacy and Pharmaceutical Sciences, University at Buffalo, USA and* [3]*Erie County Medical Center, Buffalo, New York, USA*

Abstract: The protease inhibitors are a potent, durable class of antiretroviral agents recommended as preferred initial therapy for the treatment of HIV-1 infection in combination with a nucleoside/nucleotide reverse transcriptase inhibitor. These agents play a critical role as salvage therapy in treatment-experienced patients with extensive antiretroviral drug exposure given their high genetic barrier to drug resistance. Each antiretroviral within this class is unique in virologic potency, drug-drug interaction potential, pharmacokinetic characteristics and adverse effect profile. This chapter will summarize and review protease inhibitors currently available on the market and provide guidance for the application of their use in clinical practice.

Keywords: Protease Inhibitor, Antiretroviral Therapy, Pharmacogenomics, Lopinavir, Ritonavir, Saquinavir, Darunavir, Atazanavir, Fosamprenavir, Indinavir, Nelfinavir, Tipranavir.

INTRODUCTION

The United States Department of Health and Human Sciences (DHHS) Guidelines for the Use of Antiretroviral (ARV) Agents in HIV-1 Infected Adults and Adolescents recommends nucleoside/nucleotide reverse transcriptase inhibitor (NRTI) and protease inhibitor (PI) as a preferred initial combination antiretroviral therapy (cART) regimen in treatment-naïve individuals [1]. Selection of a PI-based initial regimen may be desirable in particular patient populations at higher risk for virologic failure such as those whom adherence and proper follow-up is questioned. The goal of cART is to prevent HIV transmission, reduce morbidity and mortality through maximal virologic suppression and preservation of immune CD4+T cells and reduce CD4+ T cell activation. Despite ARV-mediated virologic suppression, HIV-positive individuals appear to have persistent T cell activation

Corresponding author Gene D. Morse: Translational Pharmacology Research Core, NYS Center of Excellence in Bioinformatics and Life Sciences, 701 Ellicott Street, Buffalo, NY 14203, USA; Tel: 716-881-7464; Fax: 716-849-6890; E-mail: qingma@buffalo.edu

when compared to HIV-uninfected comparators [2]. Ongoing T cell activation is a proposed mechanism of CD4+ T cell depletion. Sustained CD4+ T cell increases are observed in virologically suppressed individuals on cART, however, a subset of individuals fail to achieve normalized CD4+ T cells despite years of ARV treatment [2-5].

Initiation of cART during acute HIV infection has been proposed as an intervention to alter the pathogenesis and natural history of HIV infection through reduction in viral reservoirs, however, this strategy has limitations due to cumulative drug toxicities and impact on patient quality of life [6]. Introduction of early cART during acute infection introduces prolonged exposure to ARVs without known clinical benefit, medication adverse effects and risk for the development of mutant virus in the absence of strict medication adherence.

A benefit to the PI class is their potency and high genetic barrier to resistance, deeming them potentially more forgiving in instances of non-adherence. Compared to integrase strand transferase inhibitors (INSTIs), PI-associated mutations are relatively uncommon in a failing antiretroviral regimen. Resistance to protease inhibitors is dependent on both specific mutations and the number of mutations present. Head-to-head comparator trials of second-generation PIs have demonstrated similar efficacy, thus, PI selection cannot be based on efficacy alone. Each agent within this class is unique in its toxicity and tolerability profile with selection directed through clinical judgment and patient-specific characteristics. Dosing frequency, food requirements and pill burden are the factors that may contribute to non-adherence and should be considered to improve treatment outcomes [8, 9].

General PI-associated adverse effects are extensive and include gastrointestinal, metabolic, hepatic and cardiac effects [10]. Given that PIs have relatively low oral bioavailability and wide interpatient pharmacokinetic variability, most do require co-administration with the pharmacokinetic enhancer ritonavir. As the majority of PIs are substrates or inhibitors of the cytochrome P450 enzyme system, drug interactions should be a strong consideration in patients on medications metabolized through these similar pathways. Membrane transporters, specifically those belonging to the family of ATP-binding cassette transporters, affect the bioavailability and tissue penetration of protease inhibitors. P-glycoprotein (P-gp) is an efflux transporter found in the intestinal mucosa, liver, kidney, choroid plexus of the blood-brain barrier (BBB) and peripheral blood mononuclear cells (PBMCs). Protease inhibitors that inhibit P-gp also have potential to inhibit the CYP450 oxidative system thus further complicating the cascade of drug-drug interactions within this class. Presence of these transporters can impact the antiviral and toxicological activities of PIs as well their penetration to sanctuary sites undergoing active HIV replication [11].

Protease inhibitors are moderately to highly plasma protein bound, primarily to alpha-1-acid glycoprotein. Fluctuations in alpha-1-acid glycoprotein may cause significant variability in free drug concentrations. The extent of protein binding for an individual drug should be considered when determining *in vivo* inhibitory concentrations. The inhibitory quotient is defined as the trough concentration (Ctrough) divided by the 50% inhibitory concentration (IC$_{50}$] [11]. Minimum recommended target Ctrough for currently available PIs are outlined in Table **2** at the end of this chapter. Given the wide interpatient variability in plasma PI trough concentrations, therapeutic drug monitoring (TDM) has been studied to optimize clinical management of PI treatment. In treatment-experienced patients with underlying drug resistance, phenotypic information including IC$_{50}$, IC$_{90}$ and IC$_{95}$ in addition to drug concentration should be taken into consideration. Target drug concentrations are derived from phenotype interpretation with adjustment for protein binding. Ultimately, the goal is to achieve trough concentrations above the protein-binding corrected IC$_{50}$, IC$_{90}$ and IC$_{95}$. If the value obtained is below the projected range, discussion regarding medication adherence, food intake, drug-drug interactions and time of blood draw should be further investigated for intervention [12].

Although TDM is not recommended for routine use in the clinical management of HIV-infected individuals, scenarios do exist in which TDM can be considered. These instances include changes in pathophysiological states that may affect drug pharmacokinetics, pregnancy, heavily treatment-experienced individuals with reduced ARV susceptibility, concentration-dependent drug-associated toxicities, drug-drug or drug-food interactions and lack of virologic response in reported adherent individuals. Inclusion of expert opinion from clinical pharmacologists or clinical HIV pharmacy specialists within the field may be advisable to better facilitate interpretation of this information.

The protease inhibitors exhibit their antiviral effects through competitive binding at the active site of HIV protease, preventing processing of viral polyproteins, *e.g.*, gag and gag-pol. These viral polyproteins are responsible for HIV viral core maturation. The virus with an immature core which buds from the cell surface is rendered noninfectious, inhibiting further HIV viral replication and proliferation. During the late stages of the HIV life cycle, the gag-pol gene products are translated into polyproteins which eventually become immature budding particles. Protease is responsible for cleaving the precursor molecules and activating reverse transcriptase for continued viral infection. When inactivated, mature virions cannot be produced [7, 13, 14].

Availability of Approved Protease Inhibitors

Table 1. Standard dosing recommendations and drug formulations.

Protease inhibitor	Adult Dose	Formulations
Atazanavir (Reyataz)	300/100[+] mg daily (Preferred, ritonavir boosting must be used with tenofovir) 400 mg daily(PI-naïve only) 400/100 mg daily (with efavirenz naive only or tenofovir plus H_2-blocker)	150, 200, 300 mg capsule
Darunavir (Prezista)*	800/100 mg daily (Treatment-naïve and treatment-experienced with no DRV-RAM) 600/100 mg twice daily (Treatment-experienced, >1 DRV-RAM)	75, 150, 400, 600, 800 mg tablet 100 mg/ml oral suspension (strawberry)
Fosamprenavir (Lexiva)*	1400 mg twice daily (PI-naïve only) 1400/100 mg daily (PI-naïve only) 1400/200 mg daily (PI naive only); 1400/100 mg preferred [15, 16] 700/100 mg twice daily (PI-naïve or experienced)	700 mg tablet 50 mg/ml suspension (grape bubblegum peppermint)
Indinavir (Crixivan)	800 mg every 8 hours 800/100 mg twice daily	200, 400 mg capsule
Lopinavir/ritonavir (Kaletra)	400/100 mg twice daily (Treatment-experienced) 800/200 mg once daily (Treatment-naïve, <3 LPV-associated mutations)	100/25 mg, 200/50 mg tablet 80/20 mg/ml solution (cotton candy; contains 42.4% alcohol)
Nelfinavir (Viracept)	1250 mg twice daily	250, 625 mg tablet
Ritonavir (Norvir)	600 mg twice daily (Therapeutic dose, not recommended) Use limited to pharmacokinetic boosting	100 mg soft-gel capsule and tablet 80 mg/ml solution (orange, peppermint caramel)
Saquinavir	1000/100 mg twice daily	200 mg hard gel capsule 500 mg film-coated tablet
Tipranavir (Aptivus)*	500/200 mg twice daily	250 mg capsule 100 mg/ml solution (buttermint-butter toffee)

*Contains sulfonamide moiety
[+] (/100-200 mg) indicates ritonavir boosting dose

PHARMACOLOGY OF EACH OF THE APPROVED DRUGS

(Drugs are Given in Order of FDA Approval, (Fig. 1))

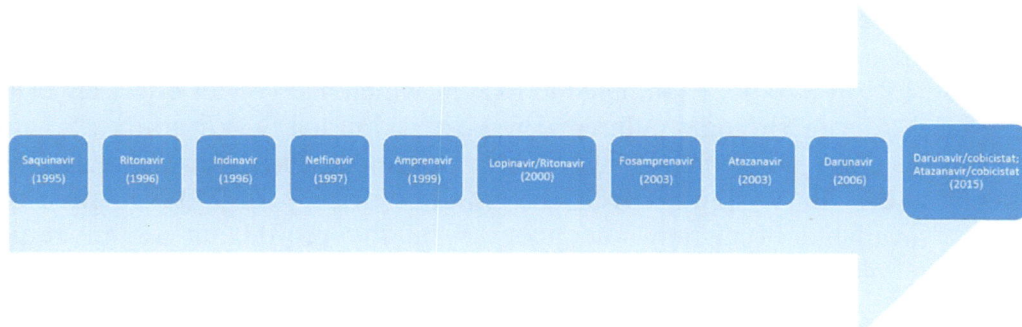

Fig. (1). Timeline of FDA-approval for protease inhibitors in the USA.

SAQUINAVIR (Invirase)

Saquinavir (SQV) was the first protease inhibitor approved by the FDA in 1995, initially marketed as saquinavir mesylate hard gelatin capsules (Invirase), and was pivotal in the movement of cART. Given the products poor oral bioavailability as an unboosted agent, a soft gelatin capsule (Fortovase) and film-coated tablet (Invirase) came to market. Today, only the SQV mesylate oral hard gel capsule and film-coated tablets are available. Saquinavir capsules require refrigeration and should be stored at 2 to 8 degrees °C. If brought to room temperature, medications are to be used within 3 months. Standard daily dosing is 1,000 mg twice daily with ritonavir (100 mg twice daily). The primary metabolic route is CYP3A4/5 with 96% excreted in the bile and 1% excreted in the urine. The primary protease inhibitor mutations which decrease susceptibility to SQV are L90M and G48V which cause a 3 and 8-fold reduction in IC_{50} [17, 18].

In October 2010, the FDA released a safety communication addressing a dose-dependent association of QT and PR interval prolongation with use of SQV recommending baseline electronic cardiogram (EKG) be performed in patients initiating therapy. Treatment is not recommended in individuals with a pre-treatment QT >450 milliseconds (ms), refractory reductions in serum hypocalcemia or hypomagnesemia, co-administration with concurrent QT-prolonging agents or in patients at risk of atrioventricular block. If EKG monitoring on treatment at day 3 or 4 indicates a QT interval > 450 ms or is > 20 ms over pre-treatment levels, discontinuation is recommended with cardiology consultation [19].

GEMINI was a 48-week, multicenter, open-label trial in treatment-naïve adults which demonstrated non-inferior virological suppression of SQV/r 1000/100 mg twice daily to LPV/r 400/100 mg twice daily. Metabolic changes were comparable between arms with the exception of triglyceride elevations which were significantly higher in the LPV/r arm (median change 14 *vs.* 55 mg/dL SQV/r *vs.* LPV/r, p=0.002) compared to SQV/r, which had greater effect on LDL cholesterol. Eleven virologic failures were observed in the SQV/r arm *vs.* 5 with LPV/r arm. One patient in the SQV/r arm developed PI-associated mutations (G48V, V82A, I84V) [20]. Given the inferior efficacy of SQV relative to currently available PI therapy and poor tolerability profile, its use in clinic practice is limited.

INDINAVIR (Crixivan)

With the advent of the HAART era, indinavir (IDV) played a pivotal role in ARV treatment; however, its use today has been replaced by more potent, less toxic PIs within the drug class. Indinavir is dosed as two 400 mg capsules every 8 hours or two 400 mg capsules every 12 hours when co-administered with 100 mg ritonavir. In HIV-positive individuals, administration with a high-fat meal was shown to effect the rate and extent of absorption by approximately 35% to 75%, an effect mitigated by co-administration with ritonavir [21]. It is recommended this agent be administered on an empty stomach (unless dosed with ritonavir) or a low-fat snack.

Indinavir undergoes metabolism primarily through CYP3A4 isoenzyme system, with approximately 11% of the dose eliminated unchanged in the urine. It is a substrate and inhibitor of CYP3A4 and inhibitor of glucuronidation. The elimination half-life is 1.8 hours, relatively unaffected by HIV status. Nephrolithiasis has been observed in approximately 10-28% of individuals receiving IDV. Risk factors include duration of treatment, patient age, fluid prophylaxis and additional RTV boosting [22]. In most instances, treatment may be continued after adequate hydration and temporary treatment interruption, however, discontinuation rates of 0.5% have been observed. Crystalluria appears to occur more commonly and may present as a spectrum of renal syndromes ranging from asymptomatic to renal stones or flank pain with or without hematuria [23]. Causes of drug crystallization include high serum levels and dehydration. Patients taking IDV should be advised to consume at least 1.5 liters of fluids (approximately 48 ounces) within 3 hours of administration to maintain urine output at $\geq$ 150 ml/hr to reduce the risk of nephrolithiasis [24]. Asymptomatic indirect hyperbilirubinemia have been observed with IDV and appear to be dose-related, typically at daily doses exceeding 2.4 grams [23]. Mucocutaneous adverse effects including paronychia, dry skin, mouth and eyes and alopecia have been observed. Alopecia may involve all hair-bearing areas with progressive regrowth after IDV discontinuation [25].

RITONAVIR (Norvir)

Today, ritonavir (RTV) is utilized primarily as a pharmacokinetic booster for other PIs at low, subtherapeutic ($\leq$ 400 mg/day) doses. When prescribed as an active PI, doses of 600 mg twice daily are used. Ritonavir is metabolized primarily through CYP3A4 and to a lesser extent CYP2D6. Ritonavir has an extensive drug-drug interaction profile as it is a substrate, inhibitor and inducer of CYP3A4, a substrate and inhibitor of P-gp, inhibitor of CYP2D6 and inducer of glucuronosyl transfer and CYP1A2 (possibly CYP2C9, CYP2C19 and CYP2B6). Literature on drug interactions is largely based on standard doses (600 mg BID) and applicability to currently prescribed daily doses is unclear. Its elimination half-life is estimated to be 3 to 5 hours [26]. Ritonavir tablets and soft-gel capsules are not bioequivalent. Relative to the soft-gel capsule, RTV tablets achieve greater maximum plasma concentrations (mean C_{max} increased 26%). Patients may experience greater adverse effects when transitioning between formulations, however, these effects are expected to diminish over time [26]

Gastrointestinal intolerance is dose-related, however, can improve with continued administration. Administration with food is not required for absorption but can improve tolerability [10, 24, 27]. Neurological disturbances including oral and peripheral paresthesia and fatigue/asthenia have been reported. Hepatotoxicity is a dose-related event with elevated risk in individuals with chronic hepatitis B or C co-infection [28]. Elevations in lipid parameters, creatine phosphokinase and uric acid as well as QTc and PR interval prolongation have been observed with RTV 400 mg twice daily [24].

NELFINAVIR (Viracept)

Given its suboptimal pharmacokinetic properties, inferior virologic efficacy and poor tolerability relative to currently available PIs, nelfinavir (NFV) is rarely utilized today in clinical practice. Nelfinavir is the only PI that is not co-administered with RTV. Oral absorption is significantly increased in the presence of food and it is recommended to be taken with food, preferably a fatty meal. In individuals with difficulty swallowing, tablets may be mixed with water and consumed immediately. The most frequently reported adverse effect with nelfinavir is diarrhea, 10-30% of cases characterized as secretory. Management can typically be handled with recommendation of inexpensive, over-the-counter remedies such as loperamide, once other infectious causes have been ruled out [29].

Nelfinavir is converted to its major metabolite hydroxyl-t-butylamide, M8 *in vitro*, which has demonstrated anti-HIV activity comparable to nelfinavir. There are at least 4 CYP enzymes involved in the metabolism of nelfinavir which include CYP3A4, CYP2C9, CYP2C19 and CYP2D6. The enzyme primarily responsible for M8 generation is CYP2C19 [30]. Nelfinavir is a substrate for CYP3A4 and CYP2C19 and inhibitor of CYP3A4 and P-gp. A genetic polymorphism of CYP2C19 has been found that may predict virologic failure in individuals exposed to NFV but its clinical relevance is unclear (Table **4**) [31]. The elimination half-life of NFV ranges from 3.5 to 5 hours with 87% (of 750 mg oral dose) removed in the feces. Urinary excretion accounts for 1-2% of the dose [30]. Nelfinavir's primary resistance mutation is D30N with associated phenotypic resistance only to NFV, not other PIs. The L90M mutation can occur which confers cross-resistance to all PIs with the exception of tipranavir and darunavir.

LOPINAVIR/RITONAVIR (Kaletra)

Lopinavir (LPV) was the first, second-generation PI available to the market and is the only PI co-formulated with RTV. Previously a twice-daily regimen, once-daily therapy (800/200 mg) is now approved in treatment-naïve individuals. The once and twice-daily regimens have been compared in treatment-naïve adults demonstrating similar virologic suppression and gastrointestinal tolerability, namely diarrhea, at 96 weeks [32]. Once-daily administration is not recommended for adults with three or more of the following LPV-associated mutations: L10F/I/R/V, K20M/N/R, L24I, L33F, M36I, I47V, G48V, I54L/T/V, V82A/C/F/S/T, and I84V [33]. LPV/r is the preferred PI in pregnancy with higher than standard doses (600/150 mg twice daily) recommended during the second and third trimesters. According to the DHHS guidelines for the initial treatment of HIV-1 infection, LPV/r (once or twice daily) with TDF/FTC or ABC/3TC is an other regimen option. Lopinavir undergoes extensive metabolism through CYP3A with less than 3% of the dose excreted unchanged in the urine. LPV/r inhibits CYP3A4 enzymes, however, based on pharmacokinetic data with amprenavir, LPV/r may be an inducer of CYP3A4 at steady state [24].

The CASTLE trial compared LPV/r 400/100 mg twice daily *vs.* ATV/r 300/100 mg once daily in 883 treatment-naïve adults. At week 96 in the ITT analysis, confirmed virologic response was observed in 74% of those in the ATV/r arm *vs.* 68% with LPV/r. In patients with a baseline CD4 <50 cells/μL (n=106), 78% response was observed with ATV/r compared to 58% with LPV/r. Higher responses were observed in ATV-treated patients with baseline HIV RNA >100,000 copies/ml. The most common adverse effect observed is gastrointestinal, primarily diarrhea occurring at moderate severity in 15-25% of patients [24]. Compared to ATV/r, significantly higher (p<0.0001) increases in fasting total cholesterol, non-HDL cholesterol and triglycerides have been observed. Mean triglyceride elevations are approximately 52 mg/dl, however, triglyceride elevations more than 700 mg/dl have been observed in approximately 4% of patients [9, 35].

ATAZANAVIR (Reyataz)

Atazanavir (ATV) is an azapeptide protease inhibitor recommended as an alternative regimen ARV therapy in treatment-naïve adults [24]. It is a preferred agent for antepartum use in combination with RTV at a dose of 300/100 mg once daily. Due to pharmacokinetic changes during the second and third trimesters, some experts recommend a dose increase to ATV/r 400/100 mg. The package insert recommends increased ATV dosing only in ARV-experienced women in the second and third trimester concurrently receiving tenofovir or an H_2 antagonist or ARV-naïve women receiving efavirenz. Atazanavir undergoes extensive metabolism through hepatic CYP3A4 with elimination primarily through the biliary route; 79% of a 400 mg dose is eliminated in the feces and 13% in the urine. In HIV-1 infected patients, the mean steady-state elimination half-life is 6.5 hours with 400 mg ATV (no ritonavir) compared to 8.6 hours with ATV/r [36]. Atazanavir is both a substrate and inhibitor of CYP3A4 and inhibitor of uridine diphosphate glucuronosyltransferase (UGT) 1A1. Absorption of ATV requires the acidic environment of the gut. Daily dose limitations to the frequently prescribed proton pump inhibitors (PPIs) are recommended in the product's package insert. In treatment-naïve adults, the maximum daily dose of omeprazole is 20 mg (equivalent to 40 mg pantoprazole, 30 mg lansoprazole) and should be administered 12 hours prior to ATV/r. Co-administration of ATV with PPIs is not recommended in treatment-experienced adults or in individuals receiving ATV without ritonavir [37, 38]. Specific dosing recommendations exist for H_2-blockers and are clearly described in the product's prescription labeling [36]. The signature mutation which confers high-level resistance to ATV is I50L. This mutation reduces ATV activity by a median of ten-fold, however, does not confer cross-resistance to other PIs including FPV which has the signature mutation I50V [24].

Reversible, clinically inconsequential increases in indirect bilirubin have been observed with ATV due to its UGT1A1 inhibitory properties. Increases in bilirubin >0.3 mg/dl may serve as surrogate markers of adherence while on ATV treatment. As previously discussed, ATV appears to have the least impact on lipid elevations or insulin resistance and has been shown to improve metabolic parameters in individuals transitioning from offending PI regimens [9, 36, 39-41]. No trials to date have compared efficacy of ATV/r to DRV/r, a first-line recommended PI, however, it appears metabolic effects of these agents are relatively comparable [42].

In a clinical trial of 1,857 patients, performed by the AIDS Clinical Trial Group (ACTG) (A5202), it was found that when comparing time to virologic failure, when ATV/r or efavirenz was given with abacavir/lamivudine or tenofovir DF/emtricitabine as initial therapy, in the abacavir–lamivudine arm the hazard ratio (HR) (efavirenz as the reference) was 1.13 (95% CI, 0.82 to 1.56). In the tenofovir DF/emtricitabine arm, the HR was 1.01 (CI, 0.70 to 1.46). Although, it was found that neither confidence interval was within the pre-specified equivalence boundaries [43]. When looking at the tolerability end point, there was a significantly longer time to modification of the 3rd drug in the regimen with ATV/r than efavirenz when both were given with abacavir and lamivudine (HR 0.69 (CI, 0.55 to 0.86) P <0.001), when given with tenofovir DF and emtricitabine a significant difference was not found (P = 0.166) [43]. Individual differences between these treatment options may be important when choosing a patient-specific regimen, and should be evaluated appropriately.

In addition, secondary outcomes from A5202 found that males and females may have altered pharmacokinetics and pharmacodynamics with ATV/r, and that the relationship between risk of viral failure and atazanavir clearance may be different between men and women [44].

In ACTG study A5257, which included 1809 patients in the final analysis, when comparing initial treatment for HIV-1 participants, it was found that raltegravir, darunavir/r and ATV/r have similar efficacy. With raltegravir being most tolerable of the three, and darunavir/r over ATV/r. However, it was mentioned that if virological failure does occur, there is less likelihood for drug resistance to develop with the ritonavir-booster protease inhibitors [45].

FOSAMPRENAVIR (Lexiva)

Fosamprenavir (FPV) is the pro-drug of its active moiety amprenavir which is rapidly converted by hydrolysis in the gut epithelium by alkaline phosphatase. Fosamprenavir has minimal antiviral activity *in vitro* and any of its antiviral activity after administration is due to amprenavir. Once absorbed, amprenavir is metabolized primarily through CYP3A4 with 75% and 14% of the dose detected as metabolites in the feces and urine [46]. Its elimination half-life is 7.7 hours. Amprenavir is both an inhibitor and inducer of CYP3A4. There are 4 FDA-approved dosing regimens which are shown in Table **1**.

Gastrointestinal intolerance including nausea, vomiting, diarrhea and abdominal pain are common and have reported in up to 40% of individuals. Diarrhea is significantly less common than with NFV [48, 49]. Rash has been observed in 12-33% of individuals exposed to FPV. FPV contains a sulfonamide moiety and the potential for cross-sensitivity between agents in the sulfonamide class is unknown. Caution should be exercised in individuals with a history of sulfa allergy with close monitoring for hypersensitivity. The ANRS-04 case control trial found FPV with or without RTV was associated with an increased risk of acute myocardial infarction (OR 1.53 per year), increased cholesterol and triglycerides. In 2009, GlaxoSmithKline (GSK) and the FDA collaboratively issued warning of this finding with addition of the claim to the product's prescribing information [50]. The I50V substitution is a common mutation associated with amprenavir exposure which decreases susceptibility to LPV and DRV.

In treatment-naïve adults, FPV demonstrated comparable virological efficacy to LPV/r in the KLEAN trial with comparable rates of gastrointestinal tolerability [52]. The ALERT trial compared once daily FPV/r (1400/100 mg) *vs.* ATV/r 300/100 mg in treatment-naïve adults. At 48 weeks in the ITT analysis, 75% and 83% achieved viral load < 50 copies/ml. Elevations in lipid parameters were similar between arms; however, triglyceride elevations were greater in those treated with FPV/r (median change 34 mg/dl *vs.* 7 mg/dl) [53].

TIPRANAVIR (Aptivus)

Tipranavir (TPV) is a novel non-peptidic protease inhibitor that retains susceptibility to virus highly resistant to other peptidomimetic protease inhibitors. In clinical practice, the use of this agent is typically reserved as salvage therapy in heavily treatment-experienced individuals with numerous PI-associated mutations. Maximal response is observed with ≤ 1 TPV-associated mutation with minimal response observed if ≥8 mutations are present. Mutations with the greatest impact on susceptibility include 74P, 47V, 58E and 82L/T. Standard dosing is 500 mg co-administered with 200 mg RTV tablets, twice daily with food to improve tolerability [54]. The elimination half-life is 6 hours. The predominant metabolic pathway involved in TPV metabolism is CYP3A4 with approximately 80% of the dose excreted in the feces and minimal urinary excretion, approximately 4% [55]. Tipranavir is a P-gp substrate and mild inhibitor, however, a potent P-gp inducer. When co-administered with RTV, a net induction in P-gp is observed despite RTV's P-gp inhibitory properties when administered alone.

Fatal and non-fatal intracranial hemorrhage (ICH) and hepatitis have been observed with TPV, each carrying a Black Box Warning for the product. Routine monitoring of coagulation parameters while receiving TPV is not currently indicated as abnormal markers have not been observed preceding ICH events. Initiation of TPV in patients at high-risk for bleeding or on concomitant antiplatelet therapy should be done with caution. The daily dose of TPV oral solution contains 1,160 IU of vitamin E which exceeds recommended allowances. Patients should be counseled to limit additional intake of vitamin E beyond that received in a standard daily multivitamin [55].

Drug discontinuation is warranted in individuals with asymptomatic elevations in AST or ALT liver enzymes greater than 10 times the upper limit of normal. AST or ALT elevations greater than 5-10 times the upper limit of normal and bilirubin levels greater than 2.5 mg/dl warrant drug discontinuation. Use of TPV is contraindicated in patients with moderate to severe (Child-Pugh B or C) hepatic impairment.

RESIST 1 and 2 compared TPV/r 500/200 mg twice daily *vs.* investigator-selected boosted PI with an optimized background regimen in treatment-experienced patients with at least 1 PI-associated primary mutation. All patients had exposure to at least 3 months of ARV therapy and to at least 3 classes of antiretroviral agents, *i.e.*, NRTI, NNRTI, and PI. Enfuvirtide was permitted in the optimized background regimen and 10% of the study group had prior exposure to the drug. Significantly more patients in the TPV/r arm achieved VL < 50 copies/ml at 48 weeks compared to comparator PI (23% *vs.* 10%, p < 0.0001).The use of enfuvirtide, baseline TPV mutation score, high TPV trough concentration, number of primary PI mutations at baseline and previous treatment with 3 or fewer PIs were found to correlate with a favorable treatment response [56].

DARUNAVIR (Prezista)

Darunavir (DRV) is a potent PI which, like TPV, retains antiviral activity against HIV strains resistant to other PIs. It is a synthetic, nonpeptidic analogue of amprenavir [14]. Darunavir is dosed once-daily in treatment-naïve and treatment-experienced individuals in the absence of DRV-associated mutations [57]. Treatment-experienced individuals with >1 DRV-associated mutation should receive 600 mg boosted with 100 mg RTV twice daily. There are no single primary mutations that confer complete resistance to DRV. The following protease inhibitor mutations are associated with reduced DRV susceptibility *in vitro* and *in vivo*: 11I, 32I, 33F, 47V, 50V, 54L/M, 73S, 74P, 76V, 84V and 89V. Darunavir is extensively metabolized through CYP3A with at least 3 oxidative metabolites, all of which are at least 10-fold less active than the parent compound against wild-type virus. Boosted-DRV has a terminal half-life of approximately 15 hours and is primarily eliminated in the feces (80%) and urine (14%) [58].

Common adverse effects (incidence ≥ 1 to <10%) include nausea, vomiting, abdominal pain, insomnia, hyperlipidemia, lipodystrophy, increased ALT, fatigue and rash [58]. Rash is usually mild to moderate in severity, occurring within 4 weeks of treatment initiation and generally resolves with continued therapy. Severe reactions including Stevens Johnson syndrome and erythema multiforme are rare and have occurred in <0.1% of individuals. Darunavir contains a sulfonamide moiety and should be avoided in individuals with severe sulfonamide allergies. Hepatotoxicity has been reported in 0.5% of individuals receiving DRV with elevated risk in individuals with underlying hepatic dysfunction such as those infected with hepatitis B or C infection [13, 31, 58]. Elevations in total cholesterol, LDL-cholesterol and triglycerides have been observed in clinical trials [58-60].

The ARTEMIS trial was a randomized, open-label study in treatment-naïve adults comparing DRV/r 800/100 mg once daily *vs.* LPV/r once or twice daily. All patients received a TDF/FTC NRTI backbone. At 96 weeks, 79% *vs.* 71% achieved VL < 50 copies/ml (p <0.001) demonstrating non-inferiority of DRV/r daily to LPV/r. Further analysis demonstrated virologic response rates in the DRV/r arm were statistically superior (p=0.012). When stratified according to baseline VL >100,000 copies/ml and CD4 cell count < 200 cells/mm^3, response rates were significantly higher with DRV/r. Lower rates of virologic failure were observed with DRV/r (12% *vs.* 17%, p=0.0437) and all virologic failures in both arms remained fully susceptible to all PIs [35]. Subgroup analyses have further shown virologic response rates are higher in DRV-treated individuals with suboptimal adherence below the suggested95% [61].

In treatment-experienced adults, twice-daily DRV/r 600/100 mg was compared to LPV/r 400/100 mg with optimized background regimen in prior virologic failures. At 96 weeks, the secondary endpoint (HIV RNA< 50 copies/ml) was 60%DRV/r *vs.* 55% with LPV/r. Grade 2-4 emergent diarrhea occurred in 8% *vs.* 15% of patients, with lesser elevations in triglycerides and total cholesterol observed with DRV/r [62]. TITAN included patients receiving ARV therapy for at least 12 weeks (LPV-naïve) of whom 47% had 3 ARV-class experience. The majority of patients (86%) had received 3 ARVs at screening with baseline susceptibility to $\geq$ 2 NRTIs (92%) and $\geq$ 4 PIs (82%) [60].

In POWER 1 and 2, treatment-experienced patients with at least 1 primary PI mutation (D30N, M46I/L, G48V, I50V/L, V82A/F/T/S, I84V, L90M) were randomized to receive DRV/r or an investigator-selected control PI regimen all with an optimized background regimen (2 or more NRTIs $\pm$ enfuvirtide). The use of NNRTIs was not permitted and TPV was not included in the control PI group as it was unavailable at time of subject enrollment [59]. Phenotypic susceptibility scores showed that 64% and 61% of DRV/r and control PI patients were resistant to all commercially available PIs (with the exception of tipranavir). Virologic response (< 50 copies/ml) was 39% for DRV/r *vs.* 9% for the control PI (p<0.001) arm [63]. These data support the role of DRV in patients with extensive antiretroviral treatment and multiclass-resistant virus.

COBICISTAT

Cobicistat (COBI) is a pharmacokinetic enhancer similar to RTV. However, unlike RTV, COBI has no intrinsic anti-HIV activity and is more selective for CYP3A potentially narrowing its drug-drug interaction profile. COBI is currently available as a co-formulated product within the single tablet regimen, Stribild (elvitegravir, cobicistat, emtricitabine, and tenofovir). It has high solubility allowing for co-formulation with currently marketed PIs, including DRV and ATV. Janssen Pharmaceuticals and Bristol-Myers Squibb received FDA approval for the first fixed-dose, combination PI regimens containing DRV and cobicistat, Prezcobix, and ATV and cobicistat, Evotaz, in January 2015 [64-66].

DRUGS IN LATE STAGES OF DEVELOPMENT

TMC310911, has been designed and developed by Tibotec Therapeutics/Janssen Therapeutics since 2005 [67]. Besides its activity against a variety of PI-resistant HIV-1 mutants as demonstrated *in vitro* [68], the potent antiviral activity of TMC310911 has been confirmed in the Phase 2 studies among treatment-naïve patients [69], with linear pharmacokinetics and a satisfactory safety profile [70]. TMC310911 is currently being evaluated as a potential drug candidate for patients with multiple PI resistance.

Table 2. HIV-1 protease inhibitor trough concentrations.

Drug	Concentration (ng/mL)
Suggested minimum target trough concentrations in patients with HIV-1 susceptible to ARV	
Fosamprenavir	400 (measured as amprenavir concentration)
Atazanavir	150
Indinavir	100
Lopinavir	1000
Nelfinavir	800
Saquinavir	100-250
Suggested minimum target trough concentrations for ART-experienced patients with HIV-1 resistant virus	
Tipranavir	20,500
Median (Range) Trough Concentration from Clinical Trials	
Darunavir (600 mg twice daily)	3300 (1255-7368)

Drug-Drug Interactions in HIV/HCV Co-infected

With the development of a new generation of hepatitis C virus (HCV) direct-acting antiviral (DAA) agents with similar efficacy in HCV mono-infected and HIV/HCV co-infected individuals, [71-73] and the risk associated with HCV complications in those with co-infection, [74, 75] the treatment of HCV in the HIV patient population has increased greatly. When treating the co-infected population for these dual infections, it is very important to be aware of drug-drug interactions to protect patients from toxicity or decreased efficacy. Many ARVs and HCV DAAs (Table **3**) have the potential for drug interactions. Depending on the "total" effect from these combined regimens, significant pharmacokinetic changes can occur.

PHARMACOGENOMICS

The pharmacogenomic investigation of protease inhibitors have focused on drug metabolism, transport, and adverse drug reactions. The findings are summarized in Table **3** and detailed information is provided in Chapter 6. Changes or mutations in genes responsible for the metabolism of these drugs have also been documented, and single nucleotide mutations associated with protease inhibitors are listed in Table **4**.

The pharmacogenomics of protease inhibitors is rather inconclusive due to conflicting findings from studies with small sample size and in general a lack of validation or confirmation. The pharmacogenomics-based precision medicine approach for protease inhibitors is promising, but warrants further investigation.

Table 3. Contains a sample of metabolic and transporter pathways of HCV DAAs Data taken from Ref. [99].

Properties	Paritaprevir [76, 77]	Ombitasvir [76, 77]	Dasabuvir [76, 77]	Asunaprevir [78-80]	Daclatasvir [81, 82]	Beclabuvir [79, 83]
Mechanism of Action	HCV NS3 protease inhibitor	HCV NS5A inhibitor	HCV NS5B non-nucleoside polymerase inhibitor	HCV NS3 protease inhibitor	HCV NS5A inhibitor	HCV NS5B non-nucleoside polymerase inhibitor
Metabolism	Substrate CYP3A4 **Inhibitor** CYP2C8 UGT1A1	Substrate CYP3A4 (minor role) **Inhibitor** CYP2C8 UGT1A1	Substrate CYP2C8 CYP3A4 CYP2D6 **Inhibitor** UGT1A1	Substrate CYP3A **Inhibitor** CYP2D6 **Inducer** CYP3A4 (weak)	Substrate CYP3A4	Substrate CYP3A4 **Inducer** CYP3A4 (weak to moderate)
Transporters	Substrate P-gp OATP1B1 OATP1B3 BCRP **Inhibitor** OATP1B1 OATP1B3 BCRP	Substrate P-gp BCRP	Substrate P-gp BCRP **Inhibitor** OATP1B1 BCRP	Substrate P-gp OATP1B1 OATP2B1 **Inhibitor** P-gp OATP1B1 (weak) OATP1B3 (weak)	Substrate P-gp **Inhibitor** P-gp OATP1B1 OCT1 BCRP	Substrate P-gp **Inhibitor** P-gp BCRP OATP1B1 OATP1B3

Table 4. Genes, single nucleoside polymorphisms (SNP), phenotypes associated with HIV-1 protease inhibitors.

Gene	SNP	Genotype	Phenotype	Function	References
CYP2C19	681G>A(*2)	Truncated protein	↑ NFV AUC; ↓ virological failure	Metabolism/response	[31, 75, 84]
CYP3A4	-392A>G(*1B)	Promoter	No effect on NFV	Metabolism	[31, 85]
CYP3A5	6986A>G(*3)	Splice defect	↓ CL/F SQV and IDV	Metabolism	[86, 87]
ABCB1	3435C>T 2677G>T	Synonymous Ala893Ser	↑ or ↓ NFV Cp, No effect on RTV, NFV, IDV	Metabolism/transport	[85, 88]

Table 4: contd...

ABCC2	-24C>T 4544G>A	Promoter Cys1515Tyr	↑ CL/F IDV; ↑ intracellular LPV	Metabolism/transport	[88, 89]
ORM1	*F1; *S		↑ CL/F of IDV; ↑ V/F of ATV	Metabolism/protein binding	[90, 91]
ApoA5	-1131T>C c.553G>T	Promoter Gly185Cys	↑ Triglycerides/cholesterol in the presence of PIs; hypertriglyceridemia in Asians	Adverse reactions	[92, 93]
ApoC3	C-482T T-455C 3238C>G (*Sst*I)	Promoter Promoter 3' UTR variant	Hyperlipidemia in the presence of RTV	Adverse reactions	[51]
ApoE	2198C>T(ε2) 2060T>C(ε4)	Arg158Cys Cys112Arg	Hyperlipidemia in the presence of RTV	Adverse reactions	[94]
CETP	-629C>A	Promoter	↑ HDL-c and non-HDL-c	Adverse reactions	[95]
TNF-α	-238G>A	Promoter	Rapid development of lipoatrophy	Adverse reactions	[47, 96]
UGT1A1	(TA)$_6$→(TA)$_7$(*28) 211G>A (*6)	Promoter; insertion Gly71Arg	Hyperbilirubinemia in presence of ATV or IDV; hyperbilirubinemia in Asians	Adverse reactions	[34, 97, 98]

CONFLICT OF INTEREST

The authors confirm that this chapter contents have no conflict of interest.

ACKNOWLEDGEMENTS

Declared none.

REFERENCES

[1]   Guidelines for the Use of Antiretroviral Agents in HIV-1-Infected Adults and Adolescents.: Department of Health and Human Services.; 2015.

[2]   Hunt PW, Martin JN, Sinclair E, *et al.* T Cell Activation Is Associated with Lower CD4+ T Cell Gains in Human Immunodeficiency Virus-Infected Patients with Sustained Viral Suppression during Antiretroviral Therapy. J Infect Dis 2003; 187(10): 1534-43.

[3]   Cohen MS, Shaw GM, McMichael AJ, Haynes BF. Acute HIV-1 infection. N Engl J Med 2011; 364(20): 1943-54.

[4]   Vinikoor MJ, Cope A, Gay CL, *et al.* Antiretroviral Therapy Initiated During Acute HIV Infection Fails to Prevent Persistent T-Cell Activation. JAIDS 2013; 62(5): 505-8 10.1097/QAI.0b013e318285cd33.

[5]   Kaufmann GR, Bloch M, Finlayson R, Zaunders J, Smith D, Cooper DA. The extent of HIV-1-related immunodeficiency and age predict the long-term CD4 T lymphocyte response to potent antiretroviral therapy. AIDS 2002; 16(3): 359-67.

[6]   Strain MC, Little SJ, Daar ES, *et al.* Effect of treatment, during primary infection, on establishment and clearance of cellular reservoirs of HIV-1. J Infect Dis 2005; 191(9): 1410-8.

[7] McDonald CK, Kuritzkes DR. Human immunodeficiency virus type 1 protease inhibitors. Arch Intern Med 1997; 157(9): 951-9.

[8] Conway B. The role of adherence to antiretroviral therapy in the management of HIV infection. J AIDS 2007; 45 Suppl 1: S14-8.

[9] Molina J-M, Andrade-Villanueva J, Echevarria J, *et al.* Once-Daily Atazanavir/Ritonavir Compared With Twice-Daily Lopinavir/Ritonavir, Each in Combination With Tenofovir and Emtricitabine, for Management of Antiretroviral-Naive HIV-1–Infected Patients: 96-Week Efficacy and Safety Results of the CASTLE Study. JAIDS 2010; 53(3): 323-32 10.1097/QAI.0b013e3181c990bf.

[10] Thiébaut R, Dabis F, Malvy D, *et al.* Serum Triglycerides, HIV Infection, and Highly Active Antiretroviral Therapy, Aquitaine Cohort, France, 1996 to 1998. JAIDS 2000; 23(3): 261-5.

[11] Catanzaro LM, Kashuba A, Corbett AH, *et al.* Protease Inhibitors (Amprenavir, Atazanavir, Indinavir, Lopinavir, Nelfinavir, Ritonavir, Saquinavir). HIV Clinical Manual 2009; Antimicrobe.org(Web): 19 Mar 2014.

[12] Acosta EP, Gerber JG. Position paper on therapeutic drug monitoring of antiretroviral agents. AIDS research and human retroviruses 2002; 18(12): 825-34.

[13] Prezista. Titusville, NJ. Janssen Therapeutics 2013; : .

[14] McCoy C. Darunavir: a nonpeptidic antiretroviral protease inhibitor. Clinical therapeutics 2007; 29(8): 1559-76.

[15] Hicks CB, DeJesus E, Sloan LM, *et al.* Comparison of once-daily fosamprenavir boosted with either 100 or 200 mg of ritonavir, in combination with abacavir/lamivudine: 96-week results from COL100758. AIDS Res Hum Retroviruses 2009; 25(4): 395-403.

[16] Cohen C, DeJesus E, LaMarca A, *et al.* Similar virologic and immunologic efficacy with fosamprenavir boosted with 100 mg or 200 mg of ritonavir in HIV-infected patients: results of the LESS trial. HIV Clin Trials 2010; 11(5): 239-47.

[17] Invirase. South San Francisco, CA. Genentech Inc 2012; : .

[18] Ananworanich J, Gayet-Ageron A, Ruxrungtham K, *et al.* Long-term efficacy and safety of first-line therapy with once-daily saquinavir/ritonavir. Antiviral Ther 2008; 13(3): 375.

[19] Communication FDS. Invirase (saquinavir) labels now contain updated risk information on abnormal heart rhythms. 2010; : .

[20] Walmsley S, Avihingsanon A, Slim J, *et al.* Gemini: A Noninferiority Study of Saquinavir/Ritonavir Versus Lopinavir/Ritonavir as Initial HIV-1 Therapy in Adults. JAIDS 2009; 50(4): 367-74 10.1097/QAI.0b013e318198a815.

[21] Zhou SY, Carver PL, Fleisher D, Kaul D, Kazanjian P, Li C. Meal Composition Effects on the Oral Bioavailability of Indinavir in HIV-Infected Patients. 1999; : .

[22] Saltel E, Angel J, Futter N, Walsh W, O'rourke K, Mahoney J. Increased prevalence and analysis of risk factors for indinavir nephrolithiasis. J Urol 2000; 164(6): 1895-7.

[23] Plosker G, Noble S. Indinavir. Drugs 1999; 58(6): 1165-203.

[24] Bartlett JG, Gallant JE, Pham PA. Medical Management of HIV Infection. Durham, NC: Knowledge Source Solutions; 2012.

[25] Bouscarat F, Prevot MH, Matheron S. Alopecia associated with indinavir therapy. N Engl J Med 1999; 341(8): 618.

[26] Norvir. North Chicago, IL. AbbVie Inc 2013; : .

[27] Bonfanti P, Valsecchi L, Parazzini F, *et al.* Incidence of Adverse Reactions in HIV Patients Treated With Protease Inhibitors: A Cohort Study. J AIDS 2000; 23(3).

[28] Sulkowski MS, Thomas DL, Chaisson RE, Moore RD. Hepatotoxicity associated with antiretroviral therapy in adults infected with human immunodeficiency virus and the role of hepatitis C or B virus infection. JAMA 2000; 283(1): 74-80.

[29] Sherman DS, Fish DN. Management of Protease Inhibitor—Associated Diarrhea. Clin Infect Dis 2000; 30(6): 908-14.

[30] Bardsley-Elliot A, Plosker G. Nelfinavir. Drugs 2000; 59(3): 581-620.

[31] Haas DW, Smeaton LM, Shafer RW, *et al.* Pharmacogenetics of long-term responses to antiretroviral regimens containing Efavirenz and/or Nelfinavir: an Adult Aids Clinical Trials Group Study. J Infect Dis 2005; 192(11): 1931-42.

[32] Gonzalez-Garcia J, Cohen D, Johnson M, *et al.* Short communication: Comparable safety and efficacy with once-daily versus twice-daily dosing of lopinavir/ritonavir tablets with emtricitabine +

tenofovir DF in antiretroviral-naive, HIV type 1-infected subjects: 96 week final results of the randomized trial M05-730. AIDS Res Hum Retroviruses 2010; 26(8): 841-5.

[33]   Kaletra. North Chicago, IL. AbbVie Inc 2013.

[34]   Rodriguez Novoa S, Barreiro P, Rendon A, *et al.* Plasma levels of atazanavir and the risk of hyperbilirubinemia are predicted by the 3435C-->T polymorphism at the multidrug resistance gene 1. Clin Infect Dis 2006; 42(2): 291-5.

[35]   Mills AM, Nelson M, Jayaweera D, *et al.* Once-daily darunavir/ritonavir vs. lopinavir/ritonavir in treatment-naive, HIV-1-infected patients: 96-week analysis. AIDS 2009; 23(13): 1679-88.

[36]   Reyataz. Princeton, NJ. Bristol-Myers Squibb Company 2013; : .

[37]   Agarwala S, Gray K, Eley T, Wang Y, Hughes E, Grasela D, editors. Pharmacokinetic interaction between atazanavir and omeprazole in healthy subjects. Program and abstracts of the 3rd IAS conference on Pathogenesis and Treatment; 2005.

[38]   Béïque L, Giguère P, La Porte C, Angel J. Interactions between protease inhibitors and acid-reducing agents: a systematic review. HIV Med 2007; 8(6): 335-45.

[39]   Johnson Ma, Grinsztejn Bb, Rodriguez Cc, *et al.* 96-week comparison of once-daily atazanavir/ritonavir and twice-daily lopinavir/ritonavir in patients with multiple virologic failures. AIDS 2006; 20(5): 711-8.

[40]   Noor MAac, Flint OPb, Maa J-Fc, Parker RAa. Effects of atazanavir/ritonavir and lopinavir/ritonavir on glucose uptake and insulin sensitivity: demonstrable differences in vitro and clinically. AIDS 2006; 20(14): 1813-21.

[41]   Nguyen ST, Eaton SA, Bain AM, *et al.* Lipid-lowering efficacy and safety after switching to atazanavir-ritonavir-based highly active antiretroviral therapy in patients with human immunodeficiency virus. Pharmacotherapy 2008; 28(3): 323-30.

[42]   Aberg JA, Tebas P, Overton ET, *et al.* Metabolic effects of darunavir/ritonavir versus atazanavir/ritonavir in treatment-naive, HIV type 1-infected subjects over 48 weeks. AIDS Res Hum Retroviruses 2012; 28(10): 1184-95.

[43]   Daar ES, Tierney C, Fischl MA, *et al.* Atazanavir plus ritonavir or efavirenz as part of a 3-drug regimen for initial treatment of HIV-1. Ann Intern Med 2011; 154(7): 445-56.

[44]   Venuto CS, Mollan K, Ma Q, *et al.* Sex differences in atazanavir pharmacokinetics and associations with time to clinical events: AIDS Clinical Trials Group Study A5202. J Antimicrob Chemother 2014; 69(12): 3300-10.

[45]   Lennox JL, Landovitz RJ, Ribaudo HJ, *et al.* Efficacy and tolerability of 3 nonnucleoside reverse transcriptase inhibitor-sparing antiretroviral regimens for treatment-naive volunteers infected with HIV-1: a randomized, controlled equivalence trial. Ann Intern Med 2014; 161(7): 461-71.

[46]   Chapman T, Plosker G, Perry C. Fosamprenavir. Drugs 2004; 64(18): 2101-24.

[47]   Maher B, Alfirevic A, Vilar FJ, Wilkins EG, Park BK, Pirmohamed M. TNF-alpha promoter region gene polymorphisms in HIV-positive patients with lipodystrophy. AIDS 2002; 16(15): 2013-8.

[48]   Gathe Jr JC, Ive P, Wood R, *et al.* SOLO: 48-week efficacy and safety comparison of once-daily fosamprenavir/ritonavir versus twice-daily nelfinavir in naive HIV-1-infected patients. AIDS 2004; 18(11): 1529-37.

[49]   Rodriguez-French A, Boghossian J, Gray GE, *et al.* The NEAT study: a 48-week open-label study to compare the antiviral efficacy and safety of GW433908 versus nelfinavir in antiretroviral therapy-naive HIV-1-infected patients. J AIDS 2004; 35(1): 22-32.

[50]   Lang S, Mary-Krause M, Cotte L, *et al.* Impact of individual antiretroviral drugs on the risk of myocardial infarction in human immunodeficiency virus–infected patients: a case-control study nested within the French Hospital Database on HIV ANRS cohort CO4. Arch Intern Med 2010; 170(14): 1228-38.

[51]   Fauvel J, Bonnet E, Ruidavets JB, *et al.* An interaction between apo C-III variants and protease inhibitors contributes to high triglyceride/low HDL levels in treated HIV patients. AIDS 2001; 15(18): 2397-406.

[52]   Eron Jr J, Yeni P, Gathe Jr J, *et al.* The KLEAN study of fosamprenavir-ritonavir versus lopinavir-ritonavir, each in combination with abacavir-lamivudine, for initial treatment of HIV infection over 48 weeks: a randomised non-inferiority trial. The Lancet 2006; 368(9534): 476-82.

[53]   Smith K, Weinberg W, DeJesus E, *et al.* Fosamprenavir or atazanavir once daily boosted with ritonavir 100 mg, plus tenofovir/emtricitabine, for the initial treatment of HIV infection: 48-week results of ALERT. AIDS Res Ther 2008; 5(1): 5.

[54]   Orman J, Perry C. Tipranavir. Drugs 2008; 68(10): 1435-63.

[55]   Aptivus. Ridgefield, CT. Boehringer Ingelheim Pharmaceuticals, Inc 2012.

[56]   Hicks CB, Cahn P, Cooper DA, *et al.* Durable efficacy of tipranavir-ritonavir in combination with an optimised background regimen of antiretroviral drugs for treatment-experienced HIV-1-infected patients at 48 weeks in the Randomized Evaluation of Strategic Intervention in multi-drug reSistant patients with Tipranavir (RESIST) studies: an analysis of combined data from two randomised open-label trials. Lancet 2006; 368(9534): 466-75.

[57]   Cahn P, Fourie J, Grinsztejn B, *et al.* Week 48 analysis of once-daily vs. twice-daily darunavir/ritonavir in treatment-experienced HIV-1-infected patients. AIDS 2011; 25(7): 929-39.

[58]   Deeks ED. Darunavir: a review of its use in the management of HIV-1 infection. Drugs 2014; 74(1): 99-125.

[59]   Clotet B, Bellos N, Molina JM, *et al.* Efficacy and safety of darunavir-ritonavir at week 48 in treatment-experienced patients with HIV-1 infection in POWER 1 and 2: a pooled subgroup analysis of data from two randomised trials. Lancet 2007; 369(9568): 1169-78.

[60]   Madruga JV, Berger D, McMurchie M, *et al.* Efficacy and safety of darunavir-ritonavir compared with that of lopinavir-ritonavir at 48 weeks in treatment-experienced, HIV-infected patients in TITAN: a randomised controlled phase III trial. Lancet 2007; 370(9581): 49-58.

[61]   Nelson M, Girard P-M, DeMasi R, *et al.* Suboptimal adherence to darunavir/ritonavir has minimal effect on efficacy compared with lopinavir/ritonavir in treatment-naive, HIV-infected patients: 96 week ARTEMIS data. J Antimicrob Chemother 2010; 65(7): 1505-9.

[62]   Banhegyi D, Katlama C, Arns da Cunha C, *et al.* Week 96 efficacy, virology and safety of darunavir/r versus lopinavir/r in treatment-experienced patients in TITAN. Curr HIV Res 2012; 10(2): 171-81.

[63]   Arastéh K, Yeni P, Pozniak A, *et al.* Short communication Efficacy and safety of darunavir/ritonavir in treatment-experienced HIV type-1 patients in the POWER 1, 2 and 3 trials at week 96. Antiviral Ther 2009; 14: 859-64.

[64]   Deeks E. Cobicistat: A Review of Its Use as a Pharmacokinetic Enhancer of Atazanavir and Darunavir in Patients with HIV-1 Infection. Drugs 2014; 74(2): 195-206.

[65]   Janssen Therapeutics. PREZCOBIX™ (darunavir/cobicistat) Approved in the US for the Treatment of Adults Living With HIV-1 2015; Retrieved from: http://www.janssentherapeutics.com/sites/default/files/pdf/PressRelease01292015.pdf.

[66]   Bristol-Myers Squibb. U.S. Food and Drug Administration Approves Bristol-Myers Squibb's Evotaz™ (atazanavir and cobicistat) for the Treatment of HIV-1 Infection in Adults [homepage on the Internet]. 2015 [April 23rd, 2015]. ; . Available from: http://news.bms.com/press-release/financial-news/us-food-and-drug-administration-approves-bristol-myers-squibbs-evotaz-a.

[67]   Surleraux DL, de Kock HA, Verschueren WG, *et al.* Design of HIV-1 protease inhibitors active on multidrug-resistant virus. J Med Chem 2005; 48(6): 1965-73.

[68]   Dierynck I, Van Marck H, Van Ginderen M, *et al.* TMC310911, a novel human immunodeficiency virus type 1 protease inhibitor, shows in vitro an improved resistance profile and higher genetic barrier to resistance compared with current protease inhibitors. Antimicrob Agents Chemother 2011; 55(12): 5723-31.

[69]   Stellbrink HJ, Arasteh K, Schurmann D, *et al.* Antiviral activity, pharmacokinetics, and safety of the HIV-1 protease inhibitor TMC310911, coadministered with ritonavir, in treatment-naive HIV-1-infected patients. J AIDS 2014; 65(3): 283-9.

[70]   Hoetelmans RM, Dierynck I, Smyej I, *et al.* Safety and pharmacokinetics of the HIV-1 protease inhibitor TMC310911 coadministered with ritonavir in healthy participants: results from 2 phase 1 studies. J AIDS 2014; 65(3): 299-305.

[71]   Rodriguez-Torres M, Gaggar A, Shen G, *et al.* Sofosbuvir for Chronic Hepatitis C Virus Infection Genotype 1-4 in Patients Coinfected With HIV. J AIDS 2015; 68(5): 543-9.

[72]   Sulkowski MS, Eron JJ, Wyles D, *et al.* Ombitasvir, paritaprevir co-dosed with ritonavir, dasabuvir, and ribavirin for hepatitis C in patients co-infected with HIV-1: a randomized trial. JAMA 2015; 313(12): 1223-31.

[73]   Osinusi A, Townsend K, Kohli A, *et al.* Virologic response following combined ledipasvir and sofosbuvir administration in patients with HCV genotype 1 and HIV co-infection. JAMA 2015; 313(12): 1232-9.

[74]   Benson CA, Kaplan JE, Masur H, Pau A, Holmes KK. Treating opportunistic infections among HIV-infected adults and adolescents: recommendations from CDC, the National Institutes of Health, and the HIV Medicine Association/Infectious Diseases Society of America. MMWR Recommendations and reports : Morbidity and mortality weekly report Recommendations and reports / Centers for Disease Control 2004; 53(RR-15): 1-112.

[75]   Di Martino V, Rufat P, Boyer N, *et al.* The influence of human immunodeficiency virus coinfection on chronic hepatitis C in injection drug users: a long-term retrospective cohort study. Hepatology 2001; 34(6): 1193-9.

[76]   Back D, editor Key Issues in Drug Interactions in the DAA era. International Conference on Viral Hepatitis (ICVH) ; 2014 ; New York, New York, USA.

[77]   Prescribing Information. Viekira Pak (paritaprevir, ritonavir, ombitasvir; dasabuvir). AbbVie Inc., North Chicago, IL. Decemeber 2014.

[78]   Garimella T AR, Stonier M, Kandoussi H, Hesney M, Colston E, Eley T, Bifano M Effect of steady-state Daclatasvir plus Asunaprevir on the single dose pharmacokinetics of the P-glycoprotein substrate digoxin in healthy adult subjects. ID Week 2014 8-12 October 2014, Philadelphia, PA, USA .

[79]   Eley T LW, Huang S-P, He B, Wang X, Chung E, Griffie A, Cooney E, Hughes EA, Kandoussi H, Sims K, Gardiner DF, Bertz RJ. Evaluation of Pharmacokinetic Drug-Drug Interactions (DDI) Between BMS-791325, an NS5b Nonnucleoside Polymerase Inhibitor, Daclatasvir, and Asunaprevir in Triple Combination in Hepatitis C Virus (HCV) Genotype 1-Infected Patients. 8th International Workshop on Clinical Pharmacology of Hepatitis Therapy, Cambridge, MA, USA, June 26–27, 2013 .

[80]   Eley T HY, Huang S, He B, Li W, Bedford W, Stonier M, Gardiner D,Sims K, Balimane P, Rodrigues D, Bertz RJ. In vivo and in vitro assessment of asunaprevir as an inhibitor and substrate of organic anion transport polypeptide (OATP) transporters in healthy volunteers [oral presentation O_04] 7th International Workshop on Clinical Pharmacology of Hepatitis Therapy, Cambridge, MA ; : .

[81]   R. B. Bristol-Myers Squibb HCV Full Development Portfolio Overview. Presented at: 14th International Workshop on Clinical Pharmacology of HIV Therapy Amsterdam, Netherlands 22-24 March 2013 .

[82]   Summary of Product Characteristics. Daklinza (daclatasvir). European Union: Bristol-Myers Squibb. October 2014 .

[83]   AbuTarif M HB, Ding Y, *et al.* The Effect of Steady-state BMS-791325, a Non-nucleoside HCV NS5B Polymerase Inhibitor, on the Pharmacokinetics of Midazolam in Healthy Japanese and Caucasian Males[Abstract P_22]. 15th International Workshop on Clinical Pharmacology of HIV and Hepatitis Therapy Washington DC, USA.

[84]   Burger DM, Schwietert HR, Colbers EP, Becker M. The effect of the CYP2C19*2 heterozygote genotype on the pharmacokinetics of nelfinavir. Br J Clin Pharmacol 2006; 62(2): 250-2.

[85]   Fellay J, Marzolini C, Meaden ER, *et al.* Response to antiretroviral treatment in HIV-1-infected individuals with allelic variants of the multidrug resistance transporter 1: a pharmacogenetics study. Lancet 2002; 359(9300): 30-6.

[86]   Anderson PL, Lamba J, Aquilante CL, Schuetz E, Fletcher CV. Pharmacogenetic characteristics of indinavir, zidovudine, and lamivudine therapy in HIV-infected adults: a pilot study. J AIDS 2006; 42(4): 441-9.

[87]   Mouly SJ, Matheny C, Paine MF, *et al.* Variation in oral clearance of saquinavir is predicted by CYP3A5*1 genotype but not by enterocyte content of cytochrome P450 3A5. Clin Pharmacol Ther 2005; 78(6): 605-18.

[88]   Colombo S, Soranzo N, Rotger M, *et al.* Influence of ABCB1, ABCC1, ABCC2, and ABCG2 haplotypes on the cellular exposure of nelfinavir in vivo. Pharmacogenet Genomics 2005; 15(9): 599-608.

[89]   Elens L, Yombi JC, Lison D, Wallemacq P, Vandercam B, Haufroid V. Association between ABCC2 polymorphism and lopinavir accumulation in peripheral blood mononuclear cells of HIV-infected patients. Pharmacogenomics 2009; 10(10): 1589-97.

[90]   Barrail-Tran A, Mentre F, Cosson C, *et al.* Influence of alpha-1 glycoprotein acid concentrations and variants on atazanavir pharmacokinetics in HIV-infected patients included in the ANRS 107 trial. Antimicrob Agents Chemother 2010; 54(2): 614-9.

[91]   Colombo S, Buclin T, Decosterd LA, *et al.* Orosomucoid (alpha1-acid glycoprotein) plasma concentration and genetic variants: effects on human immunodeficiency virus protease inhibitor clearance and cellular accumulation. Clin Pharmacol Ther 2006; 80(4): 307-18.

[92]   Chang SY, Ko WS, Kao JT, *et al.* Association of single-nucleotide polymorphism 3 and c.553G>T of APOA5 with hypertriglyceridemia after treatment with highly active antiretroviral therapy containing protease inhibitors in hiv-infected individuals in Taiwan. Clin Infect Dis 2009; 48(6): 832-5.

[93]   Guardiola M, Ferre R, Salazar J, *et al.* Protease inhibitor-associated dyslipidemia in HIV-infected patients is strongly influenced by the APOA5-1131T->C gene variation. Clin Chem 2006; 52(10): 1914-9.

[94]   Mahley RW, Rall SC, Jr. Apolipoprotein E: far more than a lipid transport protein. Annu Rev Genomics Hum Genet 2000; 1: 507-37.

[95]   Arnedo M, Taffe P, Sahli R, *et al.* Contribution of 20 single nucleotide polymorphisms of 13 genes to dyslipidemia associated with antiretroviral therapy. Pharmacogenet Genomics 2007; 17(9): 755-64.

[96]   Nolan D, Moore C, Castley A, *et al.* Tumour necrosis factor-alpha gene -238G/A promoter polymorphism associated with a more rapid onset of lipodystrophy. AIDS 2003; 17(1): 121-3.

[97]   Boyd MA, Srasuebkul P, Ruxrungtham K, *et al.* Relationship between hyperbilirubinaemia and UDP-glucuronosyltransferase 1A1 (UGT1A1) polymorphism in adult HIV-infected Thai patients treated with indinavir. Pharmacogenet Genomics 2006; 16(5): 321-9.

[98]   Rodriguez-Novoa S, Martin-Carbonero L, Barreiro P, *et al.* Genetic factors influencing atazanavir plasma concentrations and the risk of severe hyperbilirubinemia. AIDS 2007; 21(1): 41-6.

[99]   Bednasz CJ, Sawyer JR, Martinez A, *et al.* Recent advances in management of the HIV/HCV coinfected patient. Future Virology 2015; 10(8): 981-1010.

CHAPTER 6

Pharmacogenomics and Antiretroviral Therapy: Pharmacogenomics of HIV-1 Protease Inhibitors and Non-Nucleoside Reverse Transcriptase Inhibitors - Implications for Personalized Antiretroviral Therapy

Qing Ma[1,2,*], Kevin Hsu[2] and Gene D. Morse[1,2]

[1]*Translational Pharmacology Research Core, New York State Center of Excellence in Bioinformatics and Life Sciences, USA and* [2]*School of Pharmacy and Pharmaceutical Sciences, University at Buffalo, Buffalo, NY, USA*

Abstract: Recent developments in the pharmacogenomics of antiretroviral therapy have provided new prospects for the prediction of treatment efficacy and adverse effects. Current antiretroviral treatment has limitations such as high rates of adverse drug reactions and the development of resistance in a significant proportion of patients. HIV-1 protease inhibitors and non-nucleoside reverse transcriptase inhibitors are particularly suitable for genomic investigations since drug exposure/concentration and treatment response can be quantified and adverse effects can be assessed with validated measures. Additionally, there is an extensive knowledge of the pharmacokinetics of these agents, and candidate genes implicated in metabolism, transport and adverse effects have been identified. Although no unifying conclusions have been reached regarding the association of genetic variants with pharmacokinetics and adverse drug reactions, this chapter attempts to review the most recently published research and summarize the state of research in this area. Future directions for research in individualizing these agents are discussed.

Keywords: Pharmacogenomics, Personalized ART, Antiretoviral Therapy, Protease Inhibitors, Non-nucleoside Reverse Transcriptase Inhibitors, HLA-B*5701, HIV Genetics, Protease Inhibitors, NNRTI, CYP3A4/5, Hyperbilirubinemia.

INTRODUCTION

The role of pharmacogenomics is becoming increasingly important in the development of treatment algorithms to tailor patient-specific pharmacotherapy needs. HIV-1 protease Inhibitors (PI) and non-nucleoside reverse transcriptase

---

*Corresponding author Qing Ma: Translational Pharmacology Research Core, NYS Center of Excellence in Bioinformatics and Life Sciences, 701 Ellicott Street, Buffalo, NY 14203, USA; Tel: (716)881-7500; Fax: (716)849-6890; E-mail: qingma@buffalo.edu

inhibitors (NNRTI) are the integral parts of combination antiretroviral therapy (cART) in the treatment of HIV but can often be limited by their toxicity profiles. Despite their side effects, cART has significantly improved morbidity and mortality in HIV/AIDS over the past decades. However, the practice of therapy optimization can be a very challenging task. Traditional weight-based and renal/hepatic adjustment of the dosing regimen continues to produce considerable interindividual variability. The goal of pharmacogenomic testing is to limit the unpredictable pharmacokinetic profile through more individualized dosing and improve treatment response (Fig. **1**). The clinical relevance of pharmacogenomics has been demonstrated by clear relationships between *HLA-B*5701* and the type 1 hypersensitivity to abacavir and *IL28B* and treatment responses among patient with chronic hepatitis C. As a result, the risk of abacavir hypersensitivity has been effectively reduced by identifying genetic predisposition to the type 1 hypersensitivity; *IL28B* genotype-guided anti-HCV therapy significantly increases treatment success rates. The main objective of this chapter is to review the most recently published work and summarize the state of pharmacogenomics research for PIs and NNRTIs in this area. Future directions for research in individualizing these agents are also discussed.

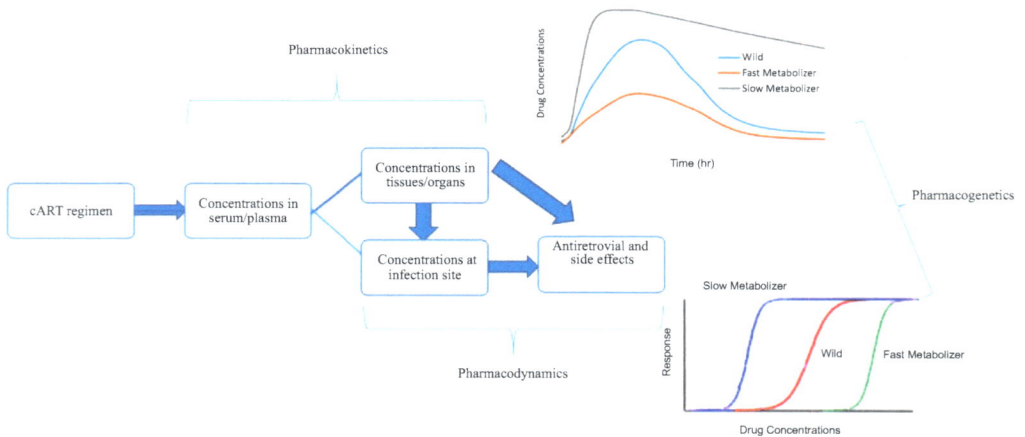

Fig. (1). Integration of pharmacokinetics, pharmacodynamics and pharmacogenetics of antiretroviral therapy.

PHARMACOGENOMICS OF PROTEASE INIHIBITORS

Cytochrome P450 Enzymes

Currently, the following PIs are commercially available: atazanavir, darunavir, fosamprenavir, indinavir, lopinavir/ritonavir, nelfinavir, saquinavir, and tipranavir. Amprenavir has been replaced by the prodrug fosamprenavir with improved bioavailability and tipranavir is only indicated for treatment-experience patients. The PIs are metabolized primarily by the cytochrome P450 (CYP) 3A enzyme subfamily into inactive metabolites except for nelfinavir, which is metabolized primarily by CYP2C19 to produce the active metabolite, M8 [1]. Ritonavir is a potent inhibitor of CYP3A enzymes and can be used to increase the bioavailability of other PIs when taken together. It also limits the pharmacokinetic variability of other PIs because of its potent inhibitory effects on CYP3A effectively producing a poor metabolizer phenotype despite the patient's genotype of the *CYP3A4/5*.

Nelfinavir is the only PI that does not require concomitant use of ritonavir as a pharmacokinetic enhancer since it does not share the same metabolic pathway as the other PIs. Variant alleles that produce a loss-of-function (LOF) in *CYP2C19* can alter the pharmacokinetic profile of nelfinavir (Table 1). The presence of the single nucleotide polymorphism (SNP) *CYP2C19* 681G>A has been associated with higher plasma nelfinavir exposure and lower M8/nelfinavir concentration ratios with the variant AA genotype [2, 3]. The presence of variant alleles in *CYP3A4/5* does not affect nelfinavir pharmacokinetics, thus suggesting that *CYP3A* enzymes might play a major role in nelfinavir disposition [3, 4].

The wild type *CYP3A5*1* genotype has been associated with an increased oral clearance of saquinavir and indinavir in contrast to variant genotypes such as the splice defect *CYP3A4*3*. [5, 6] Faster oral clearance of atazanavir was observed in *CYP3A5* expressors with the homozygous *3/*3, *6/*6, and *7/*7 alleles compared to nonexpressors, but the effect was lost with concomitant ritonavir [7]. *CYP3A4*1B* is an A to G transition at 392 basepairs upstream and may decrease protein activity due to possible disruption of the nifedipine-specific response element. It is found in 9% Caucasians and 53% African Americans but undetectable in Asian populations including Taiwanese, Chinese, or Japanese [8-10]. There is evidence that *CYP3A4*1B* is linked to the wild type *CYP3A5*1* so the phenotypic results of drug metabolism may be due to *CYP3A5*1*[11]. Haplotype analysis has linked many defective alleles with functioning alleles such as *CYP3A5*3* (splice variant) - *CYP3A4*1A* (wild-type) and *CYP3A4*16* (Thr185Ser alteration) – *CYP3A5*1E* (wild-type). [12, 13] Furthermore, *CYP3A4*16* is completely linked with the wild-type allele but not with the variant allele *CYP3A5*3*[13]. These haplotypes suggest that the presence of one LOF mutation may be compensated by another wild type allele of the CYP3A enzyme

Table 1. Genes of interest, single nucleoside polymorphisms, genotypes and phenotypes associated with combination antiretroviral therapy (modified from the reference [89])

Gene	SNP (haplotype/variant)	Genotype	Phenotype
CYP2B6	516G>T 785A>G(*4) 516 & 785 (*6) 983T>C 1459C>T(*5)	Gln172His Lys262Arg Ile328Thr Arg487Cys	↑ Cp and AUC of EFV; also associated with ↑ neurotoxicity ↑ Autoinduction of EFV in *1/*1 (wt) *vs.* *6/*6
CYP2C19	681G>A(*2)	Truncated protein	↑ NFV AUC ↓ virological failure-controversial
CYP3A4	-392A>G(*1B)	Promoter	No effect on NFV or EFV
CYP3A5	6986A>G(*3)	Splice defect	↓ CL/F of SQV and IDV
ABCB1	3435C>T 2677G>T	Synonymous Ala893Ser	↑ or ↓ NFV Cp, ↑ HDL-c with EFV, no effect on EFV autoinduction No effect on EFV, RTV, NFV, IDV
ABCC2	-24C>T 4544G>A	Promoter Cys1515Tyr	↑ CL/F of IDV with CT *vs.* CC genotype ↑ intracellular LPV in PBMC
ApoA5	-1131T>C c.553G>T	Promoter Gly185Cys	↑ Triglycerides and cholesterol in the presence of protease inhibitors Hypertriglyceridemia in Asians
ApoC3	C-482T T-455C 3238C>G (*Sst*I)	Promoter Promoter 3' UTR variant	Hyperlipidemia in the presence of RTV
ApoE	2198C>T(ε2) 2060T>C(ε4)	Arg158Cys Cys112Arg	Hyperlipidemia in the presence of RTV
CETP	-629C>A	Promoter	↑ HDL-c and non-HDL-c
HLA-DR	HLA-DRB1*0101	n/a	NVP hypersensitivity and hepatotoxicity
HLA-C	HLA-Cw-B14	n/a	NVP hypersensitivity
ORM1	*F1 *S		↑ CL/F of IDV ↑ V/F of ATV
TNF-α	-238G>A	Promoter	Rapid development of lipoatrophy
UGT1A1	$(TA)_6 \rightarrow (TA)_7$(*28) 211G>A (*6)	Promoter; insertion Gly71Arg	Hyperbilirubinemia in presence of ATV and IDV Hyperbilirubinemia in Asians

subfamily. Having both variants in *CYP3A4* and *CYP3A5* may result in the loss of genetic fitness. It is unclear what role the LOF *CYP3A4* alleles have on PI pharmacokinetics since most PIs are substrates for both *CYP3A4* and *CYP3A5*. Further investigation including haplotype analysis is warranted to determine the role of *CYP3A4* variants on PI disposition and treatment parameters. Another area of concern aside from *CYP3A* genotype is *CYP3A* expression affected by various xenobiotics and drugs. The expression may be regulated by the interaction of nuclear receptors on gene regulatory sequences or cis-acting elements. Extrinsic trans-acting elements such as pregnane X receptor (PXR) and constitutive androstane receptor (CAR) have been recognized to induce transcription *via* interactions with PXR and CAR response elements [14]. Induction of enzyme activity may lead to increased drug clearance and metabolite-induced toxicities. Genetic testing of the trans-acting elements is a possibility but this area has not provided significant clinical utility in determination of antiretroviral pharmacokinetics and treatment-related responses.

Hyperbilirubinemia

Aside from the phase I metabolic enzymes in determining drug absorption and metabolism, phase II metabolic enzymes have been associated with drug-related toxicities. Competitive inhibition of the microsomal phase II enzyme, UDP-glycuronosyltransferase (UGT) 1A1, by indinavir and atazanavir has been linked to hyperbilirubinemia and is more pronounced with the LOF allele *UGT1A1**28[15]. *UGT1A1* is involved in conjugation reactions to clear bilirubin from plasma. Two important variants have been identified as *UGT1A1**28 and *UGT1A1**6, which are associated with Gilbert's syndrome but the latter is found predominantly in South East Asians [15, 16]. The incidence of grade 3 or 4 hyperbilirubinemia is 35% whereas grade 3 or 4 elevation of aspartate aminotransferase (AST) and alanine transaminase (ALT) is 2% and 4%, respectively in clinical trials suggesting that hyperbilirubinemia is not correlated to atazanavir-induced hepatotoxicity [17]. Interestingly, there was no difference in the incidence of hyperbilirubinemia between patients with and without hepatitis B or C suggesting hepatitis status might not affect bilirubin levels.

Rodriguez-Novoa *et al.* reported that the ATP-binding cassette (ABC) polymorphism *ABCB1* 3435C>T may predict lower atazanavir trough concentrations while the wild type CC genotype predicted higher drug and bilirubin concentrations in patients receiving atazanavir containing regimen without ritonavir [18]. These findings are controversial as the role of P-glycoprotein (P-gp), the gene product of *ABCB1*, in drug disposition revealed conflicting results as other studies found association of *ABCB1* 3435C>T to neither atazanavir drug concentrations nor hyperbilirubinemia [19, 20]. Instead, Park *et al.* found an association between grade 3-4 hyperbilirubinemia to *ABCB1* 2677G>T/A and*UGT1A1**28 but could not confirm the involvement of *ABCB1* 3435C>T or *UGT1A1**6 in Koreans [20]. Adult hyperbilirubinemia is reversible and may lead to jaundice and scleral icterus which is not a severe clinical consequence; therefore, genetic testing is typically not pursued. Instead, bilirubin parameters are used as an indication of treatment adherence to atazanavir and indinavir. Variants of another class of ABC transporter *ABCC1*, *ABCC2*, and *ABCC3*, also known as the gene product multi-drug resistant protein (MRP) 1, 2, and 3, respectively, may be pursued in the neonatal population due to their role in the transport and clearance of conjugated and unconjugated bilirubin [21]. Hyperbilirubinemia will have a significant clinical impact on neonatal central nervous system as the blood-brain barrier is not fully developed [22]. However, the effect of antiretrovirals on the ABC transporters is drug specific rather than class specific and the expression of the protein is cell-specific, influenced by many factors including concomitant drugs, xenobiotics, and nuclear receptors [23]. These complex interactions will need further investigation to all possibilities. Alternatively, a one-to-one pharmacogenetic study of gene variants to the risk of hyperbilirubinemia can be pursued to investigate possible genetic associations.

ATP-Binding Cassette Transporters

Protease inhibitors are substrates of the ATP-binding cassette family of transporter P-gp. Increased P-gp expression has been shown with ritonavir, saquinavir, nelfinavir, and lopinavir in peripheral blood mononuclear cells (PBMCs) [24]. Studies of the association of PI pharmacokinetics with *ABCB1* SNPs have reported conflicting results indicating that metabolic enzymes may play a greater role in drug disposition, whereas SNPs of drug transporters may have a role in predicting treatment outcomes rather than drug disposition (Table 1). Mahungu *et al.* have discovered that the *ABCB1* 3435C>T polymorphism predicted better lipid outcomes (increased HDL-c) in patients taking efavirenz despite no association to drug concentrations [25]. In another study by Anderson *et al.* the investigators found that having at least one 2677T allele predicted greater viral suppression but not with the 3435C>T polymorphism in patients receiving indinavir without ritonavir [6].

ABCB1 3435C>T is synonymous on exon 26 that shows strong linkage disequilibrium to *ABCB1* 2677G>T/A and *ABCB1* 1236C>T. The 2677T allele is a missense mutation on exon 21 that changes the amino acid alanine to serine; the less common 2677A allele replaces the alanine with threonine. *ABCB1* 1236C>T is also synonymous located on exon 12. The most commonly studied *ABCB1* haplotype includes 1236C>T, 2677G>T, and 3435 C>T. Several studies have characterized pharmacokinetic associations to these SNP. Anderson *et al.* found that subjects with one or two copies of the wild-type CGC haplotype had lower atazanavir oral clearance consistent with previous studies that the 3435CC genotype was associated with higher atazanavir plasma concentrations without ritonavir [7, 15, 18]. Fellay *et al.* found the 3435TT genotype was associated with lower nelfinavir concentrations, lower P-gp expression in PBMC, and higher CD4+ cell counts after 6 months of therapy, while Colombo *et al.* observed higher intracellular exposure of nelfinavir with the 3435TT genotype [4, 26]. These findings suggest that the variant T allele may be less active in the efflux of nelfinavir from PBMC. However, conflicting results from various studies indicated no association between *ABCB1* genotypes and pharmacokinetics or treatment response regarding atazanavir, lopinavir/ritonavir, nelfinavir, indinavir, and saquinavir [3, 5, 19, 27]. Many of these studies included ritonavir as a pharmacokinetic enhancer and a known substrate and inhibitor of P-gp, which may partially explain the lack of genetic association [28].

Other efflux transporters include MRP and breast-cancer resistant protein (BCRP). BCRP is designated as the product of gene *ABCG2* but has not affected intracellular nelfinavir concentrations [26]. Another study indicated that PIs may act as inhibitors but not as substrates of this protein [29]. MRP is another subfamily of the ABC efflux transporter designated as the product of gene *ABCCx*. *In vivo* studies found that transgenic *ABCC2* knockout mice did not have altered lopinavir exposure but the inhibition of *ABCC2* by specific PIs is species-dependent [30, 31]. On the other hand, Elens *et al.* reported that the variant *ABCC2* 4544G>A was associated with higher PBMC intracellular lopinavir concentrations in HIV-1 infected patients [32]. Interestingly, this study did not find differences in intracellular lopinavir exposure with *CYP3A5* or*ABCB1* allelic variants. The study used the combination of lopinavir and ritonavir (400/100mg) twice daily thus the effect of ritonavir may have played a role. Colombo *et al.* were unable to confirm such an association between nelfinavir cellular exposure and genotypes of *ABCC1* or *ABCC2* [26]. Anderson *et al.* found an association between higher indinavir oral clearance and heterozygous *ABCC2* -24 CT carriers compared to the wildtype CC [6]. Since the substrate specificity to ABC transporters are agent dependent, further investigation is warranted to the more currently used PIs such as atazanavir and darunavir. However, since ritonavir is commonly used as a pharmacokinetic enhancer, it is unlikely that the genetic variations in transporters would have significant clinical relevance.

Protein Binding

Protease inhibitors are lipophilic and weakly basic making most of them highly bound to α1-acid glycoprotein [33]. Phenotypic variants of the plasma binding protein α1-acid glycoprotein, also known as orosomucoid (ORM), have shown differences in PI clearance [34, 35]. There are three variant phenotypes of *ORM1* designated as F1, F2, and S variants whereas *ORM2* is monomorphic [36]. Colombo *et al.* found that subjects with at least one copy of the F1 variant of *ORM1*had higher oral clearance of indinavir with and without ritonavir but the effect was weaker with lopinavir and not seen with nelfinavir [34]. Neither phenotypic variants nor *ORM1* plasma concentrations affected cellular concentrations of the PIs in this study. In a more recent study involving patients receiving atazanavir, the *ORM1**S phenotype was associated with increased volume of distribution [35]. The investigators noted that the moderate influence on pharmacokinetics by the S variant on atazanavir would be unlikely to have a significant clinical effect.

Metabolic Disorders

The most commonly observed adverse drug reactions associated with PI-based antiretroviral therapy are metabolic and cardiovascular disorders. The exception is atazanavir without ritonavir, which has improved profiles of triglycerides and total cholesterol after switching from the other PIs [37-41]. However, the addition of ritonavir may negate some of the lipid protective effects of atazanavir [41]. A 48-week comparative pilot study has suggested that darunavir may be as lipid friendly as atazanavir [42]. The cause of metabolic and cardiovascular disorders associated with PIs is not fully known but off-target effects on apoplipoproteins (Apo) may play an important role. Variant alleles of *ApoA-I, ApoE, and ApoC-III* can impact high-density lipoprotein (HDL-c), very-low-density lipoprotein/low-density lipoprotein (VLDL-c/LDL-c), and triglycerides, respectively. Three polymorphisms in *ApoC-III* have been associated with hypertriglyceridemia and lower HDL-c: 3238C>G (*Sst*I variant), -455T>C, and -482 C>T (Table **1**) [43, 44]. Fauvel *et al.* have compared effects of *ApoC-III* between HIV negative and positive populations and observed greater magnitude of dyslipidemia among patients with HIV infection receiving PIs thereby demonstrating that PIsmight play a strong environmental role along with the -455 variant in influencing triglycerides and HDL-c [43]. However, ethnic heterogeneity may confer lipid-protective effects despite carrying the variant *ApoC-III* alleles. Hispanics had a slight increase in triglycerides compared to Caucasians, whereas African Americans had the greatest increase [44]. *ApoE* isoforms ε2 and ε4 have been implicated to cause hypertriglyceridemia and hypercholesterolemia while the ε3 isoform is lipid-neutral [45]. Genetic variations in *ApoA5* have been associated with high triglycerides in HIV-infected subjects receiving PIs in Spain and Taiwan [46, 47]. The *ApoA5* variants -1131T>C and c.553G>T were both linked to severe hypertriglyceridemia (>500 mg/dl) [47]. Among PIs, indinavir has been significantly associated with lipodystrophy, hyperglycemia, and insulin resistance, while the use of ritonavir is linked to most lipid abnormalities [48, 49].

The mechanism for lipodystrophy is not well characterized. There are four distinct pathological disorders that constitute lipodsytrophy including lipoatrophy of subcutaneous adipose tissues of the face, limb, and buttocks; lipohypertrophy of visceral adipose tissues and subcutaneous dorsocervical adipose tissues; hyperlipidemia; and impaired glucose tolerance, insulin resistance, or diabetes mellitus. The promoter polymorphism *TNF-α* -238G>A has been associated with more rapid onset of lipoatrophy [50, 51], despite that Tarr *et al.* were unable to confirm such an association [52]. Currently, the drug tesamorelin, a growth hormone-releasing hormone synthetic analog, has been approved by the FDA in the treatment of excess abdominal fat in HIV-infected patients with lipodystrophy. Tesamorelin decreases visceral adipose tissues without reducing subcutaneous limb fat. However, this effect is not sustainable with discontinuation of the treatment; therefore, tesamorelin may not be a long-term solution for lipodystrophy even though the long-term effects of this agent on reductions in morbidity and mortality are largely unknown [53, 54]. Growth hormone and growth hormone releasing hormone (GHRH) may potentially exacerbate insulin resistance by increasing insulin-like growth factor-1 through growth hormone activation and release. Currently, there are no pharmacogenomics studies on variants of GHRH receptors or growth hormone receptors on lipid outcomes with antiretroviral therapy and require further investigation. Others genes of interest in future studies include variants of cholesterol ester transfer protein (CETP), *ABCA1*, and *ABCB1* for their role in lipid transport.

A genotype scoring system to predict dyslipidemia analogous to the Framingham 10-year cardiovascular risk assessment has been proposed to individualize antiretroviral therapy. Arnedo *et al.* have shown that the most favorable *versus* unfavorable *ApoE/ApoC3/ApoA5/CETP/ABCA1* genotypes resulted in significant differences in median triglyceride concentrations (230 mg/dl *versus* 364 mg/dl with ritonavir, 124 mg/dl *versus* 204 mg/dl without ritonavir, respectively) [55]. In regard to HDL-c, variant haplotypes of *ApoA5* contributed to lower HDL-c levels and the *CETP* -629C>A variant allele contributed to higher HDL-c levels in a gene-dose manner. The investigators also found that the homozygous variant alleles of *CETP* -629C>A (AA genotype) and endothelial lipase allele *LIPG* 584C>T (TT genotype) contributed to higher non-HDL-c levels. In all three lipid level parameters investigated, there was no gene-gene or gene-antiretroviral drug interactions. Further investigation of these lipid biomarkers and treatment response would be needed to validate such a genotype scoring system on metabolic and cardiovascular risk. Identification and analysis of polymorphic genes could tailor cART by limiting the risk of PI-related dyslipidemia and subsequent cardiovascular complications.

PHARMACOGENOMICS OF NON-NUCLEOSIDE REVERSE TRANSCRIP-TASE INHIBITORS

Cytochrome P450 Enzymes

The non-nucleoside reverse transcriptase inhibitors (NNRTIs) are noncompetitive allosteric inhibitors of HIV reverse transcriptase. The currently available NNRTIs include efavirenz (EFV), nevirapine (NVP), delavirdine (DLV), etravirine (ETR) and rilpivirine (RPV). Both efavirenz and nevirapine are primarily metabolized by CYP2B6 with minor contributions from -3A4/5 and -2A6. Delavirdine is metabolized by CYP3A4and possibly -2D6, which might be used in dual NNRTI regimens but has fallen out of preferred or alternative treatment due to its inferior efficacy. Etravirine is reserved for the treatment experienced HIV-1 infected patients with specific NNRTI mutations, which is metabolized by CYP3A4, -2C9, and -2C19. Rilpivirine is the most recent NNRTI, indicated for treatment-naïve adult patients with HIV-1 RNA less than or equal to 100,000 copies/ml, which is primarily metabolized by CYP3A.

The influence of SNPs on the pharmacokinetics and pharmacodynamics of efavirenz and nevirapine has been extensively studied (Table **1**). SNPs in *CYP2B6* have been associated with efavirenz and nevirapine drug concentrations along with their CNS toxicities. The most commonly studied SNP is *CYP2B6* 516G>T, a LOF polymorphism resulting in a glycine to histidine missense mutation that occurs frequently in African Americans (~20%) [56]. The TT variant genotype is associated with significantly decreased efavirenz clearance and increased plasma concentrations and exposure [3, 57-59]. Furthermore, the long half-life associated with the homozygous variants can increase the risk of adverse drug events due to high efavirenz exposure. Marzolini *et al.* showed that treatment failure was associated with low efavirenz concentrations while CNS side effects were more frequent in patients with high concentrations [60]. The role of *CYP2B6* 516G>T in predicting CNS side effects was limited to the first week of therapy as the adverse effects gradually resolved within 4 months of therapy, therefore, genotyping might be less predictive of long-term CNS toxicities than efavirenz concentrations [56]. Due to the long half-life and low genetic barrier of efavirenz, a concern has emerged regarding the development of resistance, particularly K103 mutation, from treatment discontinuation. Once efavirenz was discontinued, the drug persisted at low concentrations beyond 21 days in ~50% patients with the *CYP2B6* 516TT genotype [57], which might increase the development of efavirenz resistance if there is low level viremia after drug withdrawal. Studies have also examined the relationship of treatment efficacy to the *CYP2B6* 516G>T variant but no clear association was found between genotype and virologic failure or immunologic recovery [3, 56, 61].

In addition to the 516G>T polymorphism, several other LOF alleles have been identified in *CYP2B6*. 785A>G has a strong role in determining efavirenz pharmacokinetics in treatment-experienced patients [62]. However, Ribaudo *et al.* did not find any association between efavirenz concentration and 785A>G in treatment-naïve patients [57]. Another polymorphism 983T>C has been found in West African patients resulting in a complete loss-of-function leading to higher efavirenz and nevirapine plasma concentrations [63, 64]. In subjects with impaired *CYP2B6* function, accessory pathways involving *CYP2A6* and *CYP3A4/5* become increasingly important in drug metabolism. This has a significant clinical impact because the presence of LOF polymorphisms in *CYP2A6* and *CYP3A* is relatively high among different ethnic groups. Haas *et al.* have found that the *CYP3A5* 6986A>G (*3) was independently associated with efavirenz clearance [56]. Other studies have demonstrated that multiple LOF alleles at both *CYP2B6* and *CYP2A6* can produce extremely high efavirenz concentrations [65, 66]. An ~90% decrease in efavirenz elimination was observed in subjects with LOF allelic variants of *CYP2B6*, *CYP2A6*, and *CYP3A4 versus* wild type individuals [66].

*CYP2B6*variants might not only influence therapeutic efavirenz concentrations through LOF, but also affect efavirenz concentrations *via* autoinduction. Efavirenz autoinduction was initially thought to be brief, and a steady state would be reached within 6-10 days after treatment initiation [67]. However, recent studies have found that autoinduction is nonlinear and may proceed well beyond 12 weeks of therapy [68, 69]. Ngaimisi *et al.* have found a pharmacogenetic influence on efavirenz autoinduction [69]. Among the investigated SNPs in *CYP2B6*, *CYP3A5*, and *ABCB1*, the wild type of *CYP2B6* (*1/*1) had a significant influence on autoinduction: 67% of patients with *1/*1 had subtherapeutic concentrations of efavirenz (<1 µg/mL) at week 16, compared to 25% with *1/*6 and 5% poor metabolizers designated as *6/*6. This finding may impact long-term efavirenz therapy as subtherapeutic concentrations would likely lead to virologic failure and the development of resistance. The study also investigated the influence of *CYP3A5**3, *6, and *7 variants grouped together as *CYP3A5* poor metabolizers and *ABCB1* 3435C>T, which did not have a significant contribution to autoinduction. However, among the *CYP2B6* poor metabolizers, the wild-type *CYP3A5**1 allele was associated with efavirenz autoinduction suggesting a gene-gene interaction.

Nevirapine is a globally used NNRTI, particularly in resource-limited settings and remains an available ARV for cART in the United States. Similar to efavirenz, nevirapine is metabolized primarily by CYP2B6. Previous studies have confirmed the association between 516G>T polymorphism and nevirapine concentrations [59, 70, 71]. Interestingly, the 516G>T polymorphism was not able to explain variations in plasma concentrations in 50 Chinese subjects receiving nevirapine yet *CYP3A5**3 was a significant predictor in this patient population in regard to nevirapine concentrations [72]. The lack of association between 516G>T to nevirapine can be partly explained by the small sample size of patients with the TT genotype in this study. The 516TT genotype was associated with greater immunologic recovery of CD4 cells as well as decreased oral clearance of nevirapine in a pediatric cohort study [71]. Due to the small sample size of these studies, the role of *CYP2B6* in predicting nevirapine concentrations is inconclusive.

ATP-Binding Cassette Transporters

The role of the ABC transporter P-glycoprotein remains controversial for NNRTI-based therapy. Studies have reported mixed results regarding the influence of *ABCB1* polymorphisms on pharmacokinetics and treatment response with efavirenz. Efavirenz is not known to be a substrate of P-glycoprotein [73]. Yet, Fellay *et al.* have reported an association with *ABCB1* 3435C>T variants to decreased efavirenz concentrations and greater immunologic recovery at 6 months after initiation. The association to efavirenz pharmacokinetics was not replicated [3, 74, 75], nor to immunologic recovery of CD4 cells [3, 76]. Despite these conflicting reports, Haas *et al.* did find that the 3435T allele was associated with less virologic failure and less efavirenz resistance but a trend toward more toxicity-related failures [3]. In a subgroup analysis, the *ABCB1* 2677T allele was associated to less efavirenz resistance. In another study by Haas *et al.*, the 2677G>T polymorphism was associated with efavirenz exposure by univariate analysis ($p = 0.04$) [56]. Significant associations between the *ABCB1* 3435T allele and less hepatotoxicity to efavirenz and nevirapine were reported in studies with relatively small sample size [77, 78], thus need to be confirmed in a future study, as well as the contributing mechanisms.

Hypersensitivity and Hepatotoxicity

Nevirapine hypersensitivity and hepatotoxicity reactions are linked to immune reconstitution and the presence of human leukocyte antigen (HLA) gene variants. The current guidelines for the use of nevirapine restrict its use when CD4 is >250 cells/mm^3 in women and >400 cells/mm^3 in men [79]. The hypersensitivity and hepatotoxicity reactions were significantly higher with HLA-DRB1*0101 carriers and high CD4 cell counts in a Western Australian cohort [80]. This was not the case in a small Sardinian cohort [81]. Instead, the HLA-Cw-B14 haplotype was associated with nevirapine hypersensitivity despite of the small sample size (n=49). A small cohort study consisting of Japanese HIV+ patients identified the antigen HLA-Cw8 as a marker for the hypersensitivity reaction suggesting the importance of HLA-Cw8/HLA-B14 as predictors for nevirapine-associated hypersensitivity reactions in Asians [82]. The relationship between rash and hepatotoxicity during nevirapine-containing treatment remains largely unclear. The study by Martin *et al.* confirmed the association between HLA-DRB1*0101 to systemic reactions but not to isolated incidence of rash [80]. However, the incidence of rash in Caucasian patients was found to be associated with HLA-DRB1*0101 but not to CD4 percentages in patients on efavirenz or nevirapine [83]. It has been also hypothesized that P-glycoprotein might play a role in drug-related hepatotoxicity, as few studies have demonstrated an association between the *ABCB1* 3435T allele and less liver toxicity [77, 78].

Metabolic Disorders

While the majority of metabolic disorders are attributed to PI-containing cART, efavirenz-based regimens have also been associated with increased LDL-c and triglycerides (Table **1**) [84]. The mechanism is not fully understood but a number of studies have demonstrated a favorable increase in HDL-c after switching from PIs to nevirapine or efavirenz. Negredo *et al.* found that replacing PIs with nevirapine in patients with lipodsytrophy improved their lipid profiles with reductions in LDL-c and increases in HDL-c [85]. This phenomenon was partially explained by animal studies showing that nevirapine and efavirenz transiently increased HDL-c and ApoA-I production in mice [86]. The ApoA-I stimulation by nevirapine has been confirmed in 12 patients followed by HDLc increase suggesting a favorable cardiovascular profile of nevirapine [87].

The *ABCB1* variants may play an important role in predicting metabolic disorders in patients undergoing efavirenz or nevirapine containing treatments. Alonso-Villaverde *et al.* had first described the association between the 3435C>T polymorphism and changes in HDL-c concentrations in an exploratory study involving 59 HIV-infected patients over a 12 month period [88]. The wild type (CC) had the greatest increase of 36.5%, followed by 11.8% increase among the heterozygous (CT), whereas the variant (TT) did not show a significant increase. The CC also had lower serum triglycerides compared to the TT. Conversely, Mahungu *et al.* found that the TT had the greatest HDL-c increase in treatment-naïve subjects over 48 weeks [25]. The greater increase in HDL-c was also attributed to the *CYP2B6* 516TT genotype and female gender. The contribution of *ABCB1* polymorphisms to changes in lipid profiles has not been commonly studied as no physiologic mechanisms have linked P-gp to cholesterol transport. It is likely that *ABCB1*polymorphisms might serve as a surrogate for other known cholesterol efflux transporters such as ones coded by*ABCA1*.

CONCLUSION

Genetic variants continue to be associated with PI and NNRTI disposition and treatment outcomes of antiretroviral therapy. Pharmacogenomic research has identified these influences and may provide a tool for the therapeutic management of HIV infection. Currently, the risk of abacavir hypersensitivity can be effectively reduced by identifying genetic predisposition to the adverse reactions. In addition to the identification of adverse events, pharmacogenomics may have a potentially significant utility in predicting pharmacokinetics. This perhaps is one of the most powerful tools that could be clinically used to predict drug response without requiring drug assays for therapeutic drug monitoring. However, the human genome is complex. Multiple gene interactions can influence independent markers of treatment response. Further investigation of genetic variants will need to focus on a whole genome approach to capture additional gene-gene and gene-environment interactions. Pharmacogenomics might become more acceptable as a clinical test to individualize antiretroviral treatment with genomic technological advances and more clinical evidence that requires additional translational research.

CONFLICT OF INTEREST

The authors confirm that this chapter contents have no conflict of interest.

ACKNOWLEDGEMENTS

Declared none.

REFERENCES

[1]   Zhang KE, Wu E, Patick AK, *et al*. Circulating metabolites of the human immunodeficiency virus protease inhibitor nelfinavir in humans: structural identification, levels in plasma, and antiviral activities. Antimicrob Agents Chemother 2001; 45(4): 1086-93.

[2]   Burger DM, Schwietert HR, Colbers EP, Becker M. The effect of the CYP2C19*2 heterozygote genotype on the pharmacokinetics of nelfinavir. Br J Clin Pharmacol 2006; 62(2): 250-2.

[3]   Haas DW, Smeaton LM, Shafer RW, *et al*. Pharmacogenetics of long-term responses to antiretroviral regimens containing Efavirenz and/or Nelfinavir: an Adult Aids Clinical Trials Group Study. J Infect Dis 2005; 192(11): 1931-42.

[4]   Fellay J, Marzolini C, Meaden ER, *et al*. Response to antiretroviral treatment in HIV-1-infected individuals with allelic variants of the multidrug resistance transporter 1: a pharmacogenetics study. Lancet 2002; 359(9300): 30-6.

[5]   Mouly SJ, Matheny C, Paine MF, *et al*. Variation in oral clearance of saquinavir is predicted by CYP3A5*1 genotype but not by enterocyte content of cytochrome P450 3A5. Clin Pharmacol Ther 2005; 78(6): 605-18.

[6]   Anderson PL, Lamba J, Aquilante CL, Schuetz E, Fletcher CV. Pharmacogenetic characteristics of indinavir, zidovudine, and lamivudine therapy in HIV-infected adults: a pilot study. J Acquir Immune Defic Syndr 2006; 42(4): 441-9.

[7]   Anderson PL, Aquilante CL, Gardner EM, *et al*. Atazanavir pharmacokinetics in genetically determined CYP3A5 expressors versus non-expressors. J Antimicrob Chemother 2009; 64(5): 1071-9.

[8]   Ball SE, Scatina J, Kao J, *et al*. Population distribution and effects on drug metabolism of a genetic variant in the 5' promoter region of CYP3A4. Clin Pharmacol Ther 1999; 66(3): 288-94.

[9]   Sata F, Sapone A, Elizondo G, *et al*. CYP3A4 allelic variants with amino acid substitutions in exons 7 and 12: evidence for an allelic variant with altered catalytic activity. Clin Pharmacol Ther 2000; 67(1): 48-56.

[10]   Walker AH, Jaffe JM, Gunasegaram S, *et al*. Characterization of an allelic variant in the nifedipine-specific element of CYP3A4: ethnic distribution and implications for prostate cancer risk. Mutations in brief no. 191. Online. Hum Mutat 1998; 12(4): 289.

[11]   Wojnowski L, Hustert E, Klein K, *et al*. Re: modification of clinical presentation of prostate tumors by a novel genetic variant in CYP3A4. J Natl Cancer Inst 2002; 94(8): 630-1; author reply 1-2.

[12]   Saeki M, Saito Y, Nakamura T, *et al*. Single nucleotide polymorphisms and haplotype frequencies of CYP3A5 in a Japanese population. Hum Mutat 2003; 21(6): 653.

[13]   Fukushima-Uesaka H, Saito Y, Watanabe H, *et al*. Haplotypes of CYP3A4 and their close linkage with CYP3A5 haplotypes in a Japanese population. Hum Mutat 2004; 23(1): 100.

[14]   Kliewer SA, Moore JT, Wade L, *et al*. An orphan nuclear receptor activated by pregnanes defines a novel steroid signaling pathway. Cell 1998; 92(1): 73-82.

[15]   Rodriguez-Novoa S, Martin-Carbonero L, Barreiro P, *et al*. Genetic factors influencing atazanavir plasma concentrations and the risk of severe hyperbilirubinemia. AIDS 2007; 21(1): 41-6.

[16]   Boyd MA, Srasuebkul P, Ruxrungtham K, *et al*. Relationship between hyperbilirubinaemia and UDP-glucuronosyltransferase 1A1 (UGT1A1) polymorphism in adult HIV-infected Thai patients treated with indinavir. Pharmacogenet Genomics 2006; 16(5): 321-9.

[17]   Reyataz® [package insert]. Princeton, NJ: Bristol-Myers Squibb; 2010.

[18]   Rodriguez Novoa S, Barreiro P, Rendon A, *et al*. Plasma levels of atazanavir and the risk of hyperbilirubinemia are predicted by the 3435C-->T polymorphism at the multidrug resistance gene 1. Clin Infect Dis 2006; 42(2): 291-5.

[19]   Ma Q, Brazeau D, Zingman BS, *et al*. Multidrug resistance 1 polymorphisms and trough concentrations of atazanavir and lopinavir in patients with HIV. Pharmacogenomics 2007; 8(3): 227-35.

[20]   Park WB, Choe PG, Song KH, *et al*. Genetic factors influencing severe atazanavir-associated hyperbilirubinemia in a population with low UDP-glucuronosyltransferase 1A1*28 allele frequency. Clin Infect Dis 2010; 51(1): 101-6.

[21]   Bellarosa C, Bortolussi G, Tiribelli C. The role of ABC transporters in protecting cells from bilirubin toxicity. Curr Pharm Des 2009; 15(25): 2884-92.

[22]   Dennery PA, Seidman DS, Stevenson DK. Neonatal hyperbilirubinemia. N Engl J Med 2001; 344(8): 581-90.

[23]   Janneh O, Bray PG, Jones E, *et al*. Concentration-dependent effects and intracellular accumulation of HIV protease inhibitors in cultured CD4 T cells and primary human lymphocytes. J Antimicrob Chemother 2010; 65(5): 906-16.

[24]   Chandler B, Almond L, Ford J, *et al.* The effects of protease inhibitors and nonnucleoside reverse transcriptase inhibitors on p-glycoprotein expression in peripheral blood mononuclear cells in vitro. J Acquir Immune Defic Syndr 2003; 33(5): 551-6.

[25]   Mahungu TW, Nair D, Smith CJ, *et al.* The relationships of ABCB1 3435C>T and CYP2B6 516G>T with high-density lipoprotein cholesterol in HIV-infected patients receiving Efavirenz. Clin Pharmacol Ther 2009; 86(2): 204-11.

[26]   Colombo S, Soranzo N, Rotger M, *et al.* Influence of ABCB1, ABCC1, ABCC2, and ABCG2 haplotypes on the cellular exposure of nelfinavir in vivo. Pharmacogenet Genomics 2005; 15(9): 599-608.

[27]   Verstuyft C, Marcellin F, Morand-Joubert L, *et al.* Absence of association between MDR1 genetic polymorphisms, indinavir pharmacokinetics and response to highly active antiretroviral therapy. AIDS 2005; 19(18): 2127-31.

[28]   Lucia MB, Rutella S, Leone G, Vella S, Cauda R. HIV-protease inhibitors contribute to P-glycoprotein efflux function defect in peripheral blood lymphocytes from HIV-positive patients receiving HAART. J Acquir Immune Defic Syndr 2001; 27(4): 321-30.

[29]   Gupta A, Zhang Y, Unadkat JD, Mao Q. HIV protease inhibitors are inhibitors but not substrates of the human breast cancer resistance protein (BCRP/ABCG2). J Pharmacol Exp Ther 2004; 310(1): 334-41.

[30]   Ye ZW, Camus S, Augustijns P, Annaert P. Interaction of eight HIV protease inhibitors with the canalicular efflux transporter ABCC2 (MRP2) in sandwich-cultured rat and human hepatocytes. Biopharm Drug Dispos 2010; 31(2-3): 178-88.

[31]   van Waterschoot RA, ter Heine R, Wagenaar E, *et al.* Effects of cytochrome P450 3A (CYP3A) and the drug transporters P-glycoprotein (MDR1/ABCB1) and MRP2 (ABCC2) on the pharmacokinetics of lopinavir. Br J Pharmacol 2010; 160(5): 1224-33.

[32]   Elens L, Yombi JC, Lison D, Wallemacq P, Vandercam B, Haufroid V. Association between ABCC2 polymorphism and lopinavir accumulation in peripheral blood mononuclear cells of HIV-infected patients. Pharmacogenomics 2009; 10(10): 1589-97.

[33]   Bilello JA, Drusano GL. Relevance of plasma protein binding to antiviral activity and clinical efficacy of inhibitors of human immunodeficiency virus protease. J Infect Dis 1996; 173(6): 1524-6.

[34]   Colombo S, Buclin T, Decosterd LA, *et al.* Orosomucoid (alpha1-acid glycoprotein) plasma concentration and genetic variants: effects on human immunodeficiency virus protease inhibitor clearance and cellular accumulation. Clin Pharmacol Ther 2006; 80(4): 307-18.

[35]   Barrail-Tran A, Mentre F, Cosson C, *et al.* Influence of alpha-1 glycoprotein acid concentrations and variants on atazanavir pharmacokinetics in HIV-infected patients included in the ANRS 107 trial. Antimicrob Agents Chemother 2010; 54(2): 614-9.

[36]   Duche JC, Herve F, Tillement JP. Study of the expression of the genetic variants of human alpha1-acid glycoprotein in healthy subjects using isoelectric focusing and immunoblotting. J Chromatogr B Biomed Sci Appl 1998; 715(1): 103-9.

[37]   Gatell J, Salmon-Ceron D, Lazzarin A, *et al.* Efficacy and safety of atazanavir-based highly active antiretroviral therapy in patients with virologic suppression switched from a stable, boosted or unboosted protease inhibitor treatment regimen: the SWAN Study (AI424-097) 48-week results. Clin Infect Dis 2007; 44(11): 1484-92.

[38]   Mallolas J, Podzamczer D, Milinkovic A, *et al.* Efficacy and safety of switching from boosted lopinavir to boosted atazanavir in patients with virological suppression receiving a LPV/r-containing HAART: the ATAZIP study. J Acquir Immune Defic Syndr 2009; 51(1): 29-36.

[39]   Mobius U, Lubach-Ruitman M, Castro-Frenzel B, *et al.* Switching to atazanavir improves metabolic disorders in antiretroviral-experienced patients with severe hyperlipidemia. J Acquir Immune Defic Syndr 2005; 39(2): 174-80.

[40]   Nguyen ST, Eaton SA, Bain AM, *et al.* Lipid-lowering efficacy and safety after switching to atazanavir-ritonavir-based highly active antiretroviral therapy in patients with human immunodeficiency virus. Pharmacotherapy 2008; 28(3): 323-30.

[41]   Soriano V, Garcia-Gasco P, Vispo E, *et al.* Efficacy and safety of replacing lopinavir with atazanavir in HIV-infected patients with undetectable plasma viraemia: final results of the SLOAT trial. J Antimicrob Chemother 2008; 61(1): 200-5.

[42]   Aberg JA, Tebas P, Overton ET, *et al.* Metabolic effects of darunavir/ritonavir versus atazanavir/ritonavir in treatment-naive, HIV type 1-infected subjects over 48 weeks. AIDS Res Hum Retroviruses 2012; 28(10): 1184-95.

[43]   Fauvel J, Bonnet E, Ruidavets JB, *et al*. An interaction between apo C-III variants and protease inhibitors contributes to high triglyceride/low HDL levels in treated HIV patients. AIDS 2001; 15(18): 2397-406.

[44]   Foulkes AS, Wohl DA, Frank I, *et al*. Associations among race/ethnicity, ApoC-III genotypes, and lipids in HIV-1-infected individuals on antiretroviral therapy. PLoS Med 2006; 3(3): e52.

[45]   Mahley RW, Rall SC, Jr. Apolipoprotein E: far more than a lipid transport protein. Annu Rev Genomics Hum Genet 2000; 1: 507-37.

[46]   Guardiola M, Ferre R, Salazar J, *et al*. Protease inhibitor-associated dyslipidemia in HIV-infected patients is strongly influenced by the APOA5-1131T->C gene variation. Clin Chem 2006; 52(10): 1914-9.

[47]   Chang SY, Ko WS, Kao JT, *et al*. Association of single-nucleotide polymorphism 3 and c.553G>T of APOA5 with hypertriglyceridemia after treatment with highly active antiretroviral therapy containing protease inhibitors in hiv-infected individuals in Taiwan. Clin Infect Dis 2009; 48(6): 832-5.

[48]   Behrens G, Dejam A, Schmidt H, *et al*. Impaired glucose tolerance, beta cell function and lipid metabolism in HIV patients under treatment with protease inhibitors. AIDS 1999; 13(10): F63-70.

[49]   Bonnet E, Ruidavets JB, Tuech J, *et al*. Apoprotein c-III and E-containing lipoparticles are markedly increased in HIV-infected patients treated with protease inhibitors: association with the development of lipodystrophy. J Clin Endocrinol Metab 2001; 86(1): 296-302.

[50]   Nolan D, Moore C, Castley A, *et al*. Tumour necrosis factor-alpha gene -238G/A promoter polymorphism associated with a more rapid onset of lipodystrophy. AIDS 2003; 17(1): 121-3.

[51]   Maher B, Alfirevic A, Vilar FJ, Wilkins EG, Park BK, Pirmohamed M. TNF-alpha promoter region gene polymorphisms in HIV-positive patients with lipodystrophy. AIDS 2002; 16(15): 2013-8.

[52]   Tarr PE, Taffe P, Bleiber G, *et al*. Modeling the influence of APOC3, APOE, and TNF polymorphisms on the risk of antiretroviral therapy-associated lipid disorders. J Infect Dis 2005; 191(9): 1419-26.

[53]   Falutz J, Allas S, Blot K, *et al*. Metabolic effects of a growth hormone-releasing factor in patients with HIV. N Engl J Med 2007; 357(23): 2359-70.

[54]   Falutz J, Potvin D, Mamputu JC, *et al*. Effects of tesamorelin, a growth hormone-releasing factor, in HIV-infected patients with abdominal fat accumulation: a randomized placebo-controlled trial with a safety extension. J Acquir Immune Defic Syndr 2010; 53(3): 311-22.

[55]   Arnedo M, Taffe P, Sahli R, *et al*. Contribution of 20 single nucleotide polymorphisms of 13 genes to dyslipidemia associated with antiretroviral therapy. Pharmacogenet Genomics 2007; 17(9): 755-64.

[56]   Haas DW, Ribaudo HJ, Kim RB, *et al*. Pharmacogenetics of efavirenz and central nervous system side effects: an Adult AIDS Clinical Trials Group study. AIDS 2004; 18(18): 2391-400.

[57]   Ribaudo HJ, Haas DW, Tierney C, *et al*. Pharmacogenetics of plasma efavirenz exposure after treatment discontinuation: an Adult AIDS Clinical Trials Group Study. Clin Infect Dis 2006; 42(3): 401-7.

[58]   Saitoh A, Fletcher CV, Brundage R, *et al*. Efavirenz pharmacokinetics in HIV-1-infected children are associated with CYP2B6-G516T polymorphism. J Acquir Immune Defic Syndr 2007; 45(3): 280-5.

[59]   Rotger M, Colombo S, Furrer H, *et al*. Influence of CYP2B6 polymorphism on plasma and intracellular concentrations and toxicity of efavirenz and nevirapine in HIV-infected patients. Pharmacogenet Genomics 2005; 15(1): 1-5.

[60]   Marzolini C, Telenti A, Decosterd LA, Greub G, Biollaz J, Buclin T. Efavirenz plasma levels can predict treatment failure and central nervous system side effects in HIV-1-infected patients. AIDS 2001; 15(1): 71-5.

[61]   Lang T, Klein K, Fischer J, *et al*. Extensive genetic polymorphism in the human CYP2B6 gene with impact on expression and function in human liver. Pharmacogenetics 2001; 11(5): 399-415.

[62]   Lindfelt T, O'Brien J, Song JC, Patel R, Winslow DL. Efavirenz plasma concentrations and cytochrome 2B6 polymorphisms. Ann Pharmacother 2010; 44(10): 1572-8.

[63]   Mehlotra RK, Bockarie MJ, Zimmerman PA. CYP2B6 983T>C polymorphism is prevalent in West Africa but absent in Papua New Guinea: implications for HIV/AIDS treatment. Br J Clin Pharmacol 2007; 64(3): 391-5.

[64]   Wyen C, Hendra H, Vogel M, *et al*. Impact of CYP2B6 983T>C polymorphism on non-nucleoside reverse transcriptase inhibitor plasma concentrations in HIV-infected patients. J Antimicrob Chemother 2008; 61(4): 914-8.

[65]   di Iulio J, Fayet A, Arab-Alameddine M, *et al*. In vivo analysis of efavirenz metabolism in individuals with impaired CYP2A6 function. Pharmacogenet Genomics 2009; 19(4): 300-9.

[66]   Arab-Alameddine, M., *et al*., Pharmacogenetics-based population pharmacokinetic analysis of efavirenz in HIV-1-infected individuals. Clin Pharmacol Ther, 2009. **85**(5): p. 485-94.

[67]   Barrett JS, Joshi AS, Chai M, Ludden TM, Fiske WD, Pieniaszek HJ, Jr. Population pharmacokinetic meta-analysis with efavirenz. Int J Clin Pharmacol Ther 2002; 40(11): 507-19.

[68]   Zhu M, Kaul S, Nandy P, Grasela DM, Pfister M. Model-based approach to characterize efavirenz autoinduction and concurrent enzyme induction with carbamazepine. Antimicrob Agents Chemother 2009; 53(6): 2346-53.

[69]   Ngaimisi E, Mugusi S, Minzi OM, *et al*. Long-term efavirenz autoinduction and its effect on plasma exposure in HIV patients. Clin Pharmacol Ther 2010; 88(5): 676-84.

[70]   Penzak SR, Kabuye G, Mugyenyi P, *et al*. Cytochrome P450 2B6 (CYP2B6) G516T influences nevirapine plasma concentrations in HIV-infected patients in Uganda. HIV Med 2007; 8(2): 86-91.

[71]   Saitoh A, Sarles E, Capparelli E, *et al*. CYP2B6 genetic variants are associated with nevirapine pharmacokinetics and clinical response in HIV-1-infected children. AIDS 2007; 21(16): 2191-9.

[72]   Chen J, Sun J, Ma Q, *et al*. CYP2B6 polymorphism and nonnucleoside reverse transcriptase inhibitor plasma concentrations in Chinese HIV-infected patients. Ther Drug Monit 2010; 32(5): 573-8.

[73]   Stormer E, von Moltke LL, Perloff MD, Greenblatt DJ. Differential modulation of P-glycoprotein expression and activity by non-nucleoside HIV-1 reverse transcriptase inhibitors in cell culture. Pharm Res 2002; 19(7): 1038-45.

[74]   Winzer R, Langmann P, Zilly M, *et al*. No influence of the P-glycoprotein genotype (MDR1 C3435T) on plasma levels of lopinavir and efavirenz during antiretroviral treatment. Eur J Med Res 2003; 8(12): 531-4.

[75]   Motsinger AA, Ritchie MD, Shafer RW, *et al*. Multilocus genetic interactions and response to efavirenz-containing regimens: an adult AIDS clinical trials group study. Pharmacogenet Genomics 2006; 16(11): 837-45.

[76]   Winzer R, Langmann P, Zilly M, *et al*. No influence of the P-glycoprotein polymorphisms MDR1 G2677T/A and C3435T on the virological and immunological response in treatment naive HIV-positive patients. Ann Clin Microbiol Antimicrob 2005; 4: 3.

[77]   Haas DW, Bartlett JA, Andersen JW, *et al*. Pharmacogenetics of nevirapine-associated hepatotoxicity: an Adult AIDS Clinical Trials Group collaboration. Clin Infect Dis 2006; 43(6): 783-6.

[78]   Ritchie MD, Haas DW, Motsinger AA, *et al*. Drug transporter and metabolizing enzyme gene variants and nonnucleoside reverse-transcriptase inhibitor hepatotoxicity. Clin Infect Dis 2006; 43(6): 779-82.

[79]   Panel on Antiretroviral Guidelines for Adults and Adolescents. Guidelines for the use of antiretroviral agents in HIV-1-infected adults and adolescents : Department of Health and Human Services; January 10, 2011 [cited 2011 February 17]. ; . Available from: http://www.aidsinfo.nih.gov/ContentFiles/AdultandAdolescentGL.pdf.

[80]   Martin AM, Nolan D, James I, *et al*. Predisposition to nevirapine hypersensitivity associated with HLA-DRB1*0101 and abrogated by low CD4 T-cell counts. AIDS 2005; 19(1): 97-9.

[81]   Littera R, Carcassi C, Masala A, *et al*. HLA-dependent hypersensitivity to nevirapine in Sardinian HIV patients. AIDS 2006; 20(12): 1621-6.

[82]   Gatanaga H, Yazaki H, Tanuma J, *et al*. HLA-Cw8 primarily associated with hypersensitivity to nevirapine. AIDS 2007; 21(2): 264-5.

[83]   Vitezica ZG, Milpied B, Lonjou C, *et al*. HLA-DRB1*01 associated with cutaneous hypersensitivity induced by nevirapine and efavirenz. AIDS 2008; 22(4): 540-1.

[84]   Squires K, Lazzarin A, Gatell JM, *et al*. Comparison of once-daily atazanavir with efavirenz, each in combination with fixed-dose zidovudine and lamivudine, as initial therapy for patients infected with HIV. J Acquir Immune Defic Syndr 2004; 36(5): 1011-9.

[85]   Negredo E, Ribalta J, Paredes R, *et al*. Reversal of atherogenic lipoprotein profile in HIV-1 infected patients with lipodystrophy after replacing protease inhibitors by nevirapine. AIDS 2002; 16(10): 1383-9.

[86]   Tohyama J, Billheimer JT, Fuki IV, Rothblat GH, Rader DJ, Millar JS. Effects of nevirapine and efavirenz on HDL cholesterol levels and reverse cholesterol transport in mice. Atherosclerosis 2009; 204(2): 418-23.

[87]   Franssen R, Sankatsing RR, Hassink E, *et al*. Nevirapine increases high-density lipoprotein cholesterol concentration by stimulation of apolipoprotein A-I production. Arterioscler Thromb Vasc Biol 2009; 29(9): 1336-41.

[88]   Alonso-Villaverde C, Coll B, Gomez F, *et al*. The efavirenz-induced increase in HDL-cholesterol is influenced by the multidrug resistance gene 1 C3435T polymorphism. AIDS 2005; 19(3): 341-2.

[89]   Owen A, Pirmohamed M, Khoo SH, Back DJ. Pharmacogenetics of HIV therapy. Pharmacogenet Genomics 2006; 16(10): 693-703.

CHAPTER 7

HIV Co-Treatment

Sarah Nanzigu[1,*], Jaran Eriksen[2] and Pauline Byakika-Kibwika[3]

[1]*Department of Pharmacology and Therapeutics, College of Health Science, Makerere University, Uganda;* [2]*Department of Laboratory Medicine, Division of Clinical Pharmacology, University Hospital at Huddinge, Karolinska Institutet, Sweden and* [3]*Department of Medicine, College of Health Sciences, Makerere University, Uganda*

Abstract: The roll-out of life saving antiretroviral medication has improved the quality of life and increased the life expectancy of HIV-infected individuals. HIV-infected individuals suffer more ailments compared to the general population, necessitating frequent co-medications. There is considerable geographic overlap between areas with high prevalence of HIV and other infectious diseases such as malaria, tuberculosis, and neglected tropical diseases raising the possibility of complex polypharmacy and drug-drug interactions. The cytochrome P450 (CYP450) enzymes play a major role in metabolism of many of the ARVs and drugs used for the treatment of other prevalent diseases; thus co-treatment creates potential for CYP450 mediated drug interactions. Some ARVs pose a particularly high-risk for potential drug-drug interactions, which may be pharmacokinetic or pharmacodynamic in nature and can result in raising or lowering plasma or tissue concentrations of co-prescribed drugs. Elevated drug concentrations may be associated with drug toxicity and lower drug concentrations may be associated with therapeutic failure. This chapter provides an in-depth understanding of clinically relevant drug-drug interactions during treatment of HIV and common illnesses and reviews the currently available data on interactions between ARVs and drugs used in the management of some other common illnesses.

Keywords: HIV/ART, Concomitant Treatment, AIDS-related Diseases, Co-treatments, HAART, drug interactions, NNRTI, CYP540, HIV and Cancer, HIV and Malaria, Rifampicin.

INTRODUCTION

Antiretroviral therapy (ART) is often co-administered with several other medications owing to frequent occurrence of AIDS-related diseases (ARDs). Some diseases including malaria, tuberculosis and AIDS related cancers tend to share geographical distribution with HIV, and their prevalence and/or severity is increased by HIV infection [1-4]. Furthermore, patients on HAART today have a

---

*Corresponding author Sarah Nanzigu: Department of Pharmacology and Therapeutics, Makerere University College of Health Sciences, Uganda; Tel: 256784843045; Fax: 256414532947;
E-mails: snanzigu@yahoo.com; snanzigu@chs.mak.ac.ug

life expectancy close to that of HIV negative persons, which leads to an increasing proportion of patients that also need treatment for *e.g.* hypertension and hyperlipidemia. HIV itself, as well as some ARVs also have an increased risk of hyperlipidemia. This makes co-treatment a frequent occurrence with potential for drug interactions in the HIV infected population [1, 4]. For purposes of addressing the need in regions with high HIV prevalence, this chapter will mostly address interactions with the WHO recommended first and second-line ART whose summary also appear in the Appendix of this chapter.

Most of the antiretroviral drugs, especially the non-nucleoside reverse transcriptase inhibitors (NNRTI) and the protease inhibitors (PI) are metabolized by the cytochrome P450 (CYP450) group of enzymes. Some drugs induce while others inhibit function of these enzymes [5]. The CYP450 group of enzymes is subdivided into families and sub-families each catalysing the metabolism of different drugs. The CYP3A sub-family plays the biggest role in the metabolism of drugs, including ARVs, and it is mostly at this level that drug-drug interactions arise [6]. Other pathways involving uridine diphosphate glucuronyl transferases (UGT), membrane transport proteins such as P-glycoprotien (Pgp), organic anion-transporting polypeptides (OATP) and organic cation proteins (OCT) also play a role in the pharmacokinetics of drugs [7] and therefore have a role in drug-drug interactions. Studies showed dual upregulation of the CYP3A4/ P-gp by some drugs, predicting dual CYP3A4/ P-gp drug-drug interactions [8].

Pharmacology of Reverse Transcriptase Inhibitors (RTIs) Relevant to Drug Interactions

Nucleoside Reverse Transcriptase Inihibitors (NRTIs)

The NRTIs including zidovudine, lamivudine, zalcitabine, didanosine, and emtricitabine require three steps of intracellular phosphorylation to the active 5' triphosphate form [9-13]. Competetion for the phosporylation process by drugs in this group has been reported, limiting co-administration for some of these agents [9-11]. Zalcitabine (ddc) significantly inhibits the phosphorylation of lamivudine (3TC) and zidovudine (AZT) [9, 10], and plasma concentrations of AZT and stavudine (d4T) may be significantly reduced during co-adminstration with 3TC or didanosine (ddi) [14]. Although some NRTIs including lamivudine and emtricitabine are excreted unchanged in urine thus posing minimal potential for CYP450 mediated interactions, most of the drugs in this class are substrates of the phase II conjugation reactions catalysed by enzymes that include grucoronyl transferase and alcohol dehydrogenase [12]. Therefore co-administration of NRTI with drugs that interfere with phosphorylation, phase II conjugation reactions or share the same excretory pathway may lead to significant interactions.

Nucleotide Reverse Transcriptase Inhibitor (NtRTI)

This class of drugs including tenofovir require two steps of intracellular phosphrylation to the active diphosphate form [13, 15]. Data on competition by NtRTI for the phosphorylation process is limited. Co-administration with some of the NTRIs such as emtricitabine (FTC) is safe. The NtRTIs are primarily excreted through tubular secretion [16]. Tenofovir is a substrate of the P-gp (ABCB1/MDR1) and Breast Cancer Resistance Protein (ABCG2/BCRP) [17]. PIs exhibit a dose dependant inhibition of the intestinal P-gp hence increase absorption and plasma concentrations of tenofovir [18, 19].

Neither NRTIs nor NtRTIs are metabolized by CYP450 enzymes thus pose no risk for CYP mediated interactions with other drugs. Nonetheless, some of the frequently co-administered antimcrobial agents, may affect phase II metabolism, influencing pharmacokinetics of NRTIs.

Non-Nucleoside Reverse Transcriptase Inhibitors (NNRTIs)

The NNRTIs include efavirenz, nevirapine, delavirdine, etravirine and rilpivirine. Unlike the NRTIs, NNRTIs neither need intracellular phosphorylation nor do they interfere with this process [20, 21]. However, NNRTIs are largely metabolized by CYP450 enzymes, mainly the CYP3A4 and CYP2B6, with some of the agents having the ability to induce or inhibit these enzymes [7, 22]. The NNRTIs therefore pose higher risk for drug interactions. Efavirenz, the most widely used NNRTI, is mainly catalysed by CYP2B6, assisted by CYP3A5, CYP1A2 and CYP3A4 [23, 24]. The action of additional enzymes; CYP2A6, CYP2C19 is also observed at increasing efavirenz concentrations [23-25]. Both efavirenz and nevirapine show a time dependant induction of the activity of enzymes responsible for their own metabolism, so-called auto induction [25-28]. This is due to the drugs' strong ability to activate the human constitutive androgenic receptor (hCAR) and human pregnane X receptor (hPXR) that are key transcription regulators of the CYP2B6 and CY3A4 [29, 30]. The activation of these receptors result in a time and perhaps dose dependant induction of the CYP2B6 and 3A4 enzymes [25, 31-33]. Efavirenz also induces CYP2C19, CYP3A5, UGT2B7, and ABCB1 [7, 25, 32, 34, 35]. Data also indicate a gene-dependant enzyme induction of CYP2B6, UGT2B7 and CYP2C19 by efavirenz, with fast metabolising genotypes exerting a more extensive enzyme induction [25, 32, 34-36]. The effect of efavirenz on CYP3A4 and 2C19 may be mixed with instances of initial inhibition followed by induction. Efavirenz also has minimal inhibition of CYP1A2, 2C9 and 2D6 [7, 37].

Efavirenz has been shown to up-regulate several drug transporters including ABCB1, ABCG2, ABCC2, ABCC3, ABCC5, ABCG2, ABCC1, ABCC4, ABCC5, and SLCO3A1 and SLCO2B1 [38]. It is is therefore one of the drugs that can cause dual drug-drug interaction with substrates of the CYP450 and their drug transporters [8, 38]. However, efavirenz has not been shown to induce intestinal CYP3A4 and P-gp, which may indicate hepatic specific enzyme induction of CYP450 by this drug [39].

Nevirapine is primarily metabolized by CYP3A4 and CYP2B6 with minor involvement of CYP3A5, 2C9, 2C19, 2A6 and 2D6, followed by glucuronidation of the hydroxylated metabolites [40-73]. Like efavirenz, nevirapine strongly induces the CYP3A4, CY2B6 and 2C9 mainly through hCAR activation [44], but so far the drug is only shown to inhibit the CYP3A4-mediated 10-hydroxylation of warfarin at concentrations that are beyond therapeutic relevance [41]. Nevirapine is a substrate of the multi resistance protein 7 (MRP7) also known as ABCC10, which is also a transporter for tenofovir, zalcitabine and nucleoside analogues used in cancer chemotherapy [45-47].

Etravirine shares many properties with efavirenz including the mixed inhibition and induction profiles. Etravirine is metablised by CYP3A4, 2C9, 2C19 and metabolites undergo glucuronidation [48]. It induces CYP3A4, CYP2B6 and UGT, but inhibits CYP2C9, 2C19 and the P-glycoprotein [7, 48].

Rilprivirine is metabolized by CY3A4, CYP2C19, CYP1A2, with minor assistance from CYP2C8, 2C9 and 2C10 [7, 49]. It is a weak inducer of CYP3A4, CYP2B6 and 2C19, but may inhibit CYP2B6 and CYP1A2.

Pharmacology of Protease Inhibitors (PIs) Relevant to Drug Interactions

Generally, PIs including ritonavir (RT), lopinavir (LPV), indinavir (IDV), nelfinavir (NFV), amprenavir (AMPV), and saquinavir (SQV) are metabolized by CYP3A4 and they express varrying potential to inhibit this isoenzyme with ritonavir having the greatest inhibitory effect [50]. Three protease inhibitors; RT, IDV and NFV are classified as strong CYP3A4/5 inhibitors causing more than 80% reduction in clearance or at least 5 fold increase in AUC of CYP3A4 substrates [51]. Ritonavir has the highest potency for hepatic and intestinal CYP3A4 inhibition, causing up to 80% reduction in hepatic activity of the

CYP3A group of enzymes, and it is primarily used as a pharmacokinetic booster of antiviral drugs that are substrates of CYP3A [52-55]. Indinavir, and nelfinavir follow ritonavir in potency of hepatic CYP3A4 inhibition, while saquinavir is considered less potent [52, 53]. Ritonavir and saquinavir inhibit both CYP3A4 and CYP3A5 while nelfinavir inhibits all the CYP3A group of enzymes [53]

Ritonavir shows a mixed profile towards CYP3A4 and CYP2D6; induction with short term administration and strongly inhibiting the CYP3A4 and CYP2D6 enzyme with chronic administration [7, 52, 55]. Ritonavir and nelfinavir can also weakly inhibit the fetal CYP3A7 isoenzyme [53]. Ritonavir has the ability to induce CYP1A2, CYP2C9, 2C19, P-gp and UGT, and may inihibit CYP2C9 [55].

Nelfinavir is metabolized by CPY2C19 in addition to CYP3A4 but is shown to only inhibit the CYP3A group of enzymes. Amprenavir, atazanavir and lopinavir also inhibit the CYP3A4 insoenzymes to different extents [56].

Pharmacology of Entry Inhibitors Relevant to Drug Interactions

The CCR5 receptor antagonist maraviroc is metabolized by CYP3A4/5, and is a substrate of P-gp [57]. Therefore co-adminstration with CYP3A4 inhibitors has been shown to increase maraviroc exposure while CYP3A4 inducers reduce its exposure.

Pharmacology of Integrase Inhibitors (INSTI) Relevant to Drug Interactions

The integrase inhibitors raltegravir and dolutegravir primarily undergo glucuronidation UGT1A1, assisted by UGT1A3 and UGT1A9. Elvitegravir is primarily metabolized by CYP3A4/5 assisted by UGT1A1. Integrase inhibitors are substrates of the p-gp but they neither induce nor inhibit CYP450 group of enzymes and transporters.

INTERACTIONS OF ANTIRETROVIRAL AGENTS AND TREATMENTS FOR COMMON ILLNESSES

Although availability and use of ARVs may differ depending on resources, selection of a suitable HAART regimen from readily available ARVs may be influenced by concurrent infections. Generally, the World Health Organization (WHO) currently advises an NNRTI based regimen in combination with two NRTIs (preferably TDF+FTC or 3TC+ABC with EFV) as first line and PI based regimen in combination with two NRTIs as second line in resource limited settings [58, 59]. Regimens are selected on individual basis in resource rich settings [58]. This general rule may not apply in the face of co-infections and drug-drug interactions necessitating adjustments in the selection of specific ARVs. However, use of fixed dose combination regimens limits individualisation of regimens, especially in resource limited settings.

INTERACTIONS BETWEEN ARVs AND TREATMENTS FOR HEPATITIS C AND B

Infection with hepatitis C virus (HCV) among HIV patients is around 25% in parts of Europe, warranting good understanding of drug-drug interactions during HIV-HCV management [60, 61]. Compared to HCV monoinfection, treating HVC/HIV co-infected patients is complicated by a poorer immunity, drug-interactions, overlaping toxicities and poor adherence to treatment [62]. Treatment of chronic HCV with ribavirin (RBV) and pegylated interferon-alpha (Peg-IFN) both of which enhance host clearance of HCV showed success in HIV-HCV co-infected persons [63]. However, toxicity and strong bidirectional drug-drug interactions are among the reported limitations [64]. Ribavirin inhibits the phosphorylation of NRTI increasing the risk of virological failure in poorly monitored HIV patients. There may also be increased risk of hematological toxicity during zidovudine and ribavirin co-administration [64]. Ribivirin and didanosine co-administration is contraindicated due to a high risk of hepatic failure following increased intracellular concentrations of ddi [64]. Abacavir may reduce plasma levels of ribavirin but no effect has been seen on HCV virological response [63, 65, 66].

In an attempt to improve efficacy and safety in HCV treatments, drugs that directly disrupt viral replication by inhibiting specific nonstructural proteins of the virus, the directly actying antiviral agents (DAAs) were developed. These drugs are classied according to the non-structural protein they target: inhibitors of NS3/4A protease, NS5A protein, or NS5B polymerase [67]. There are several DAAs, including those approved and those that are still undergoing clinical trials: The first generation DAAs, boceprevir and telaprevir, both of which are HCV NS3/4A protease inhibitors, were in 2011 approved for treating HCV, including genotype-1 infection, with each of these drugs used in combination with Peg-IFN and RBV [68, 69]. Boceprevir, an inhibitor of HCV NS3/4A protein is metabolized by CYP3A4/5 with contribution of aldo-keto reductase while telaprevir is primarily metabolized by CYP3A4 [69, 70]. Both NS3/A4 inhibitors are substrates of the P-gp and they strongly inhibit CYP3A4 and the P-gp, which may cause increased exposure of primary CY3A4 substrates [71]. However, both drugs reduce the plasma exposure of ritonavir boosted atazanavir and darunavir, and likewise, the plasma concentrations of both boceprevir and telaprevir are reduced during co-administration with ritonavir boosted HIV PIs and efavirenz [71, 72]. Although the mechanisms are poorly understood, an increase in the proportion of unbound drugs during co-adminstration with darunavir suggests a protein displacement interaction between these drugs and HIV protease inhibitors. Therefore, co-administration of these first generation HCV PIs with ritonavir boosted PI is not recommended, except for telaprevir and ATV/r.

Telaprevir may be co-administered with efavirenz under close monitoring and dosage adjustment but boceprevir and efavirenz co-administration is not recommended in some settings [58, 71]. Zidovudine, didanosine, nevirapine co-administration should be avioded due to increased risks of toxicity during HCV treatment with ribavirin-PegIFN/ Ribavirin treatment [58]. These two HCV PIs are thought to induce CYP2C19, reducing plasma exposure of its primary substrates necessitating adjustment of telaprevir dose [71].

Newer generation DAAs including; simeprevir, sofosbuvir, ledipasvir, daclatasvir, grazoprevir, elbasvir and faldaprevir, show much better efficacy and safety profiles, and are thought to be less prone to drug-drug interactions during HCV and HCV-HIV co-treatment [73-76]. Simeprevir, an HCV NS3/4A protease inhibitor and, the HCV NS5B polymerase inhibitor sofsbuvir, were in 2013 approved for combined or inteferon-free treatments of HCV, following evidence of better efficacy, tolerability and adherence compared to RBV, Peg-Info and first generation DAAs [69, 73, 77]. These newer generation DDAs are not completely spared of drug-drug interactions. Simeprevir is an HCV NS3/4A protease inhibitor, a substrate of CYP3A4, and inhibitor of intestinal CYP3A4 and hepatic CYP1A29. Co-adminsitration of simeprevir and NNRTI (efavirenz, delavirdine, etravirine and nevirapine) may lead to bidirectional reduction in plasma concentrations of both simeprevir and NNRTIs, and 71% reduction in the plasma exposure of simeprevir was observed during efavirenz co-administration [78, 79]. On the other hand, interactions between simeprevir and protease inhibitors can lead to bidirection increase on concentrations of either simeprevir and the Pis. Plasma exposure of simeprevir was increased by 2.6 folds following coadministration with ritonavir boosted dalunavir, accompanied by 32% increase in ritonavir exposre. Therefore, efavirenz, darunavir and ritovir boosted PIs are not recommeneded for coadministration with simeprevir [78]. No significant changes have been observed during coadministration of simeprevir with tenofovir, rilpivirine and raltegravir. Maraviroc and INSTI-based HAART regimens may therefore be preffered during HCV co-treatment with simeprevir [78, 79].

The incidence of infection with hepatitis B virus (HBV) among HIV patients is up to 30% in sub-Saharan Africa (SSA), but treatment of HIV-HBV co-infected patients is less complicated given the availability of ARVs with antiHBV activity [58, 80]. This allows for the selection of HAART combinations including drugs that act against both viruses such as TDF, FTC and 3TC. Adefovir and entecavir are alternative NRTIs when tenofovir is not safe [58]. Adefovir undegoes the same phosphorylation process as tenofovir, and is excreted unchanged in urine [81]. Adefovir may increase the plasma concentrations and toxicity of tenofovir and other ARVS that are excreted unchanged; hence, co-administration is not recommended [64].

INTERACTIONS BETWEEN ARVs AND TREATMENTS FOR MALARIA

The geographical overlap in the epidemiology of Malaria and HIV infections creates significant disease interactions. HIV increases risk, incidence and severity of malaria while malaria increases HIV viral replication and viral load in HIV-infected individuals [82-84]. Poor response to malaria treatment may be observed in either treated or untreated HIV infected patients [85, 86]. The poor malaria treatment response is due to the low immunity caused by HIV and possibly the drug-drug interactions between ARVs and antimalarial drugs [84, 87, 88]. The current WHO malaria treatment guidelines for uncomplicated falciparum malaria recommend use of artemisinin based combination therapy (ACTs) [89] such as *artemether* plus lumefantrine (AL), *dihydroartemisinin* plus piperaquine (DHA + PPQ), *artesunate* plus either amodiaquine, or mefloquine, or sulfadoxine-pyrimethamine

Recommended drugs for the treatment of severe malaria include parenteral artesunate as first–line, with quinine and artemether as alternatives. Following parenteral antimalarial therapy and resumption of oral intake, therapy is completed with a a full course of an ACT.

Artemether and artesunate, are primarily metabolized by CYP3A4 and CYP2B6, with ability to induce CYP3A4, CYP2B6, CYP2C19 and the P-gp, but inhibit CYP1A2 [90-95]. Specifically, artemether is metabolized to its metabolite dihydroartemisinin by CYP2B6, assisted by CYP3A4, CYP2A6, and UGT1A1, and it induces CYP3A4 and CYP2B6 [90, 93]. Artesunate is metabolized by CYP2A6 to its metabolite dihydroartemisinin. Dihydroartemisinin undergoes glucuronidation by UGT1A9 and UGT2B6 [93]. Artemether, artesunate and their metabolite dihydroartemisinin (DHA) are all active against malaria. Lumefantrine is primarily metabolized by CYP3A4 and it inhibits CYP2D6 [90]. The major players in the metabolism of ACT; CYP3A4, CYP2B6, CYP2A6, and UGT are the same enzymes that are involved in the metabolism of most ARVs, and hence, clinically relevant drug-drug interactions may occur during the treatment of malaria-HIV co-infected patients [88, 90, 93]. Strong induction or inhibition of the CYP3A4, CYP2A6/B6 and other contributing enzymes can greatly influence concentration and therapeutic outcomes [88]. The following have been observed:-

Clinically Relevant Interactions

- Efavirenz induces CYP2B6, CYP3A4 and UGT1A, leading to increased clearance of artemerther, DHA and lumefanfrine, and significant reduction in their plasma exposure.

- Delavidine inhibits CYP3A4, CYP2C9 and CYP2C19 leading to increased toxicity of lumefantrine, artemether and halofantrine [84].

- PIs, most especially ritonavir boosted lopinavir, inhibit CYP3A4 leading to reduced clearance of the ACTs [52-56, 96], but no clinically significant effect on treatment outcome.

Possibly due to the above interactions and the inherent antimalarial potential of protease inhibitors [96], better malaria treatment outcomes were observed when ACTs were co-administered with ritonavir-boosted lopinavir than with NNRTI based ART [87, 97]. Even though ACTs induce enzymes involved in the clearance of ARVs, the clinical relevance of this interaction is questionable. Nonethelsess, the following interactions have been reported:

- Artemether induces CYP3A4, leading to increased clearance of nevirapine and significantly reducing its plasma exposure while efavirenz is not significantly affected, and,

- Nevirapine, efavirenz and artemesinins exhibit time and dose dependant induction of their own metabolism.

- Nevirapine induces CYP3A4 and CYP2B6, increasing the clearance of artemether and DHA, lowering their plasma exposure but with no significant effects on lumefantrine.

Amodiaquine is metabolized by both hepatic and extra-hepatic CYP2C8, CYP1A1 and CYP1B1and it is known to inhibit CYP2C6 and CYP2C9 [98, 99]. Mefloquine is metabolized by CYP3A4 and the drug has no known effects on

CYP450 group of enzymes [100]. Piperaquine is also primarily metabolized by CYP3A4 with contribution from CYP2C8 [101]. Quinine is a substrate of P-gp, metabolized by CYP3A4/5 with some involvement of 2C19, 2C9, 2D6 and CYP 1A2, and also undergoes glucuronidation [102-105]. Quinine and primaquine induce CYP1A1/2, and quinine inhibits CYP2D6 but the clinical importance of this has not been studied [106]. The following have been observed:

- NNRTIs significantly reduced the plasma exposure and may affect therapeutic outcomes of quinine through the induction of CYP3A4/5, while PIs reduce the metabolism of quinine by inhibiting these enzymes [107, 108]. While co-administration with NNRTI may reduce the efficacy of quinine, protease inhibitors may increase its toxicity.

- Co-administration of amodiaquine and efavirenz led to increased hepatotoxicity

- Co-administration of amodiaquine with zidovudine containing ARV regimen lead to marked neutropenia

- Concomitant use of amodiaquine and CYP2C8 inhibitors including ritonavir, lopinavir and saquinavir is not advised [109]. Inducers of CYP3A4 like the NNRTI and rifampicin may reduce plasma levels of mefloquine and piperaquine while PIs may increase their exposure and toxicity [100]

Commonly used agents in travelers for chemoprophlaxis against malaria include atovaquone which undergoes glucuronidation, and proguanil which is metabolized by CYP2C8. Efavirenz, lopinavir and ritonavir have been shown to reduce plasma concentrations of both atovaquone and proguanil through increased glucuronidation and CYP2C8 activity [110].

INTERACTIONS BETWEEN ARVS AND TREATMENTS FOR MYCOBACTERIA TUBERCULOSIS

The HIV prevalence among TB infected patients is as high as 50% in SSA and South America making HIV-TB co-treatment considerations especially important in these regions. The first line antimycobacterial agents include rifamycins (rifampicin and rifabutin), isoniazid, pyrazinamide and ethambutol. Other drugs including streptomycin, clarithromycin, ciprofloxacin may be used in the second line. Through the induction of the CYP450 enzymes, efavirenz, nevirapine and rifampicin increase their own clearance and that of co-administered drugs [111, 112]. Rifampicin is the greatest known CYP450 inducer of both hepatic and intestinal CYP enzymes including CYP3A4/5, CYP2A6, CYP2B6, CYP1A2, CYP2C8/9 and CYP2C18/19; and the P-gp [111, 112]. This results in increased metabolism of several drugs including efavirenz, nevirapine, maraviroc and PIs [112]. The commonly co-administered antituberculosis agents, isoniazid and pyrazinamide, have been shown to inhibit accessory pathways involved in the metabolism of NNRTI, with isoniazid having the greatest inhibitory effect [113, 114]. Co-administration of rifampicin with efavirenz showed reduced exposure of efavirenz [115-118]. Rifampicin has been shown to reduce the bioavaliability and plasma levels of maraviroc through the induction of CYP3A4 and p-gp, and increasing maraviroc dosage to 600mg daily has been recommended during maraviroc and rifampicin co-administration. Rifampicin also induces UGT enzymes and has been shown to increase the clearance of zidovudine. Rifabutin interacts to a much smaller extent, and can therefore be used as an alternative to rifampicin. However, the drug is expensive and currently not much used in low-income settings.

INTERACTIONS BETWEEN ARVS AND CANCER TREATMENTS

The prevalence of both AIDS-related and non-AIDS related cancers has increased during the HIV epidemic [119, 120], and is higher among HIV infected individuals than in the general population, making the topic of cancer and HIV co-treatment very important [121]. Seropositivity of karposis sarcoma herpes virus among HIV infected individuals is up to 50% in some African settings, while non-Hodgkin's lymphomas are the second commonest AIDS related cancers in Africa [122-124]. Bi-directional drug interactions and verlapping toxicities are observed during management of cancer patients who are co-infected with HIV.

There following overlapping toxicities between HAART and anticancer agents need to be considered with cancer chemotherapy taking precedence over HAART [125]:-

- Platinums, taxanes, and vinca-alkaloids frequently cause peripheral neuropathy, and hence co-administration with ARVs with the same side effects, including didanosine and stavudine should be avoided.

- ARVs with myelosuppressant effects like zidovudine and cancer agents with similar effects including cyclophosphamide should be avoided or co-administered with caution.

- Anthracyclines, arsenic trioxide, dasatinib, lapatinib, nilotinib, sunitinib and tamoxifen are associated with QT prolongation and co-administration with PIs with overlapping toxicities including atazanavir, ritonavir-boosted lopinavir and saquinavir should be avoided [125].

Modification of CYP450 activity by NNRTI and Protease inhibitors may increase concentrations and toxicity of some anticancer agents, while some anticancer agents interfere with CYP450 enzymes increasing concentrations and toxicity of NNRTIs and Pis [126]. The vinca alkaloids including vincristine, vimblastine and semisynthetic vinca alkaloid vinirelbine, that are commonly used agents for kaposis sarcoma, and Tyrosine kinase inhibitors are substrates of the CYP3A4 [127, 128], predicting clinically relevant interactions with both CYP3A4 inducers like efavirenz and inhibitors like the protease inhibitors. The texane anticancer agent paclitaxel is similar to vinca alkaloids, and strongly induces CYP3A4 through activation of the hPXR [129]. The alkylating agent cyclophosphamide requires CYP2B6 and CYP2C19 to form the active metabolites, that are metabolized by CYP3A4 to inactive and potentially neurotoxic metabolites. This leads to the following clinically significant interactions:

- CYP2C19 inhibitors like etravrine may reduce production of the active metabolite of cyclophosphamide, affecting anticancer therapuetic outcomes [126]

- NNRTIs induce CYP2B6 leading to over production of the active metabolite leading to possible cyclophosphamide toxicity [126].

- CYP3A4 inibitors including protease inhibitors, elvitegravir and cobistat may reduce metabolism of cyclophosphamide increasing chances of toxicity of the anticancer agent [126].

Dosage adjustments should be considered during co-administration of the above agents [128]. Dexamethasone is a substrate and concentration-dependent inducer of CYP3A4 hence, prolonged co-administration may lower concentration of protease inhibitors [128].

Drug-drug interactions exist during HIV cotreatment with non infectious disease including and drugs used in cardiovacrular conditions and antihyperlipidemic drugs. However, this chapter concentrated on interactions between HAART and treatment for infectious diseases.

CONFLICT OF INTEREST

The authors confirm that this chapter contents have no conflict of interest.

ACKNOWLEDGEMENTS

Declared none.

REFERENCES

[1]   Herrero MD, Rivas P, Rallon NI, Ramirez-Olivencia G, Puente S. HIV and malaria. AIDS Rev. 2007; 9(2): 88-98.

[2]   Akinbo FO, Omoregie R. Plasmodium falciparum infection in HIV-infected patients on highly active antiretroviral therapy (HAART) in Benin City, Nigeria. J Res Health Sci 2012; 12(1): 15-8.

[3]   Tuberculosis and HIV [homepage on the Internet]. UCSF; c2013. Available from: http: //hivinsite.ucsf.edu/InSite?page=kb-05-01-06#S2X/

[4]   AIDS.Gov. Tuberculosis and HIV [homepage on the Internet]. [updated: 14 November 2013; cited: 20th May 2014]. Available from: http: //www.aids.gov/hiv-aids-basics/staying-healthy-with-hiv-aids/potential-related-health-problems/tuberculosis/

[5]   Walubo A. The role of cytochrome P450 in antiretroviral drug interactions. Expert opinion on drug metabolism & toxicology 2007; 3(4): 583-98.

[6]   The human cytochrome P450 (CYP) allele nomentclature database [homepage on the Internet]. [updated 2013; cited: 05th August 2013]. Available from: http://www.cypalleles.ki.se/

[7]   Rathbun RC, Liedtke MD. Antiretroviral drug interactions: overview of interactions involving new and investigational agents and the role of therapeutic drug monitoring for management. Pharmaceutics 2011; 3(4): 745-81.

[8]   Schuetz EG, Beck WT, Schuetz JD. Modulators and substrates of P-glycoprotein and cytochrome P4503A coordinately up-regulate these proteins in human colon carcinoma cells. Mol Pharm 1996; 49(2): 311-8.

[9]   Morris GW, Laclair DD, McKee EE. Pyrimidine deoxynucleoside and nucleoside reverse transcriptase inhibitor metabolism in the perfused heart and isolated mitochondria. Antiviral Ther 2010; 15(4): 587-97.

[10]   Kewn S, Veal GJ, Hoggard PG, Barry MG, Back DJ. Lamivudine (3TC) phosphorylation and drug interactions *in vitro*. Biochem Pharmacol 1997; 54(5): 589-95.

[11]   Durand-Gasselin L, Da Silva D, Benech H, Pruvost A, Grassi J. Evidence and Possible Consequences of the Phosphorylation of Nucleoside Reverse Transcriptase Inhibitors in Human Red Blood Cells. Antimicrob Agents Chemother 2007; 51(6): 2105-11.

[12]   Masho SW, Wang CL, Nixon DE. Review of tenofovir-emtricitabine. Ther Clin Risk Manag 2007; 3(6): 1097-104.

[13]   Piliero PJ. Pharmacokinetic properties of nucleoside/nucleotide reverse transcriptase inhibitors. J Acquir Immune Defic Syndr 2004; 37 Suppl 1: S2-s12.

[14]   Note R, Maisonneuve C, Lettéron P, *et al.* Mitochondrial and Metabolic Effects of Nucleoside Reverse Transcriptase Inhibitors (NRTIs) in Mice Receiving One of Five Single- and Three Dual-NRTI Treatments. Antimicrob Agents Chemother 2003; 47(11): 3384-92.

[15]   Fung HB, Stone EA, Piacenti FJ. Tenofovir disoproxil fumarate: a nucleotide reverse transcriptase inhibitor for the treatment of HIV infection. Clin Ther 2002; 24(10): 1515-48.

[16]   Munoz de Benito RM, Arribas Lopez JR. Tenofovir disoproxil fumarate-emtricitabine coformulation for once-daily dual NRTI backbone. Expert review of anti-infective therapy 2006; 4(4): 523-35.

[17]   Neumanova Z, Cerveny L, Ceckova M, Staud F. Interactions of tenofovir and tenofovir disoproxil fumarate with drug efflux transporters ABCB1, ABCG2, and ABCC2; role in transport across the placenta. AIDS 2014; 28(1): 9-17.

[18]   Tong L, Phan TK, Robinson KL, *et al.* Effects of human immunodeficiency virus protease inhibitors on the intestinal absorption of tenofovir disoproxil fumarate *in vitro*. Antimicrob Agents Chemother 2007; 51(10): 3498-504.

[19]   Mwafongo A, Nkanaunena K, Zheng Y, *et al.* Renal events among women treated with tenofovir/emtricitabine in combination with either lopinavir/ritonavir or nevirapine: analysis from the AIDS Clinical Trial Group A5208 trial. AIDS 2014.

[20]   Drake SM. NNRTIs—a new class of drugs for HIV. J Antimicrob Chemother 2000; 45(4): 417-20.

[21]   Smith PF, DiCenzo R, Morse GD. Clinical pharmacokinetics of non-nucleoside reverse transcriptase inhibitors. Clin Pharmacokinet 2001; 40(12): 893-905.

[22]   Ma Q, Okusanya OO, Smith PF, *et al.* Pharmacokinetic drug interactions with non-nucleoside reverse transcriptase inhibitors. Expert opinion on drug metabolism & toxicology 2005; 1(3): 473-85.

[23]   Arab-Alameddine M, Di Iulio J, Buclin T, *et al.* Pharmacogenetics-based population pharmacokinetic analysis of efavirenz in HIV-1-infected individuals. Clin Pharmacol Ther 2009; 85(5): 485-94.

[24]   Ward BA, Gorski JC, Jones DR, Hall SD, Flockhart DA, Desta Z. The cytochrome P450 2B6 (CYP2B6) is the main catalyst of efavirenz primary and secondary metabolism: implication for HIV/AIDS therapy and utility of efavirenz as a substrate marker of CYP2B6 catalytic activity. J Pharmacol Exp Ther 2003; 306(1): 287-300.

[25]   Nanzigu S. Host Variabilities Influencing HIV/ART Outcomes, Scholars' Press; 2013. Available from: http://www.amazon.com/Host-Variabilities-Influencing-Outcomes-Pharmacokinetics/dp/3639702190/

[26]   Kappelhoff BS, van Leth F, MacGregor TR, Lange J, Beijnen JH, Huitema AD. Nevirapine and efavirenz pharmacokinetics and covariate analysis in the 2NN study. Antiviral Ther 2005; 10(1): 145-55.

[27]   Nanzigu S, Eriksen J, Makumbi F *et al.* Pharmacokinetics of the nonnucleoside reverse transcriptase inhibitor efavirenz among HIV-infected Ugandans. HIV Med 2012; 13(4): 193-201.

[28]   Zhu M, Kaul S, Nandy P, Grasela DM, Pfister M. Model-Based approach to characterize efavirenz autoinduction and concurrent enzyme induction with carbamazepine. Antimicrob Agents Chemother 2009; 53(6): 2346-53.

[29]   Faucette SR, Zhang TC, Moore R, *et al.* Relative activation of human pregnane X receptor *versus* constitutive androstane receptor defines distinct classes of CYP2B6 and CYP3A4 inducers. Journal of Pharmacol Exp Ther 2007; 320(1): 72-80.

[30]   Habtewold A, Amogne W, Makonnen E, Yimer G, Nylen H, Riedel KD, *et al.* Pharmacogenetic and pharmacokinetic aspects of CYP3A induction by efavirenz in HIV patients. Pharmacogenomics J 2013; 13(6): 484-9.

[31] Robertson SM, Maldarelli F, Natarajan V, Formentini E, Alfaro RM, Penzak SR. Efavirenz induces CYP2B6-mediated hydroxylation of bupropion in healthy subjects. J Acquir Immune Defic Syndr 2008; 49(5): 513-9.

[32] Ngaimisi E, Mugusi S, Minzi OM, *et al*. Long-term efavirenz autoinduction and its effect on plasma exposure in HIV patients. Clin Pharmacol Ther 2010; 88(5): 676-84.

[33] Hariparsad N, Nallani SC, Sane RS, Buckley DJ, Buckley AR, Desai PB. Induction of CYP3A4 by efavirenz in primary human hepatocytes: comparison with rifampin and phenobarbital. J Clin Pharmacol 2004; 44(11): 1273-81.

[34] Michaud V, Kreutz Y, Skaar T, *et al*. Efavirenz-mediated induction of omeprazole metabolism is CYP2C19 genotype dependent. Pharmacogenomics 2013.

[35] Habtewold A, Amogne W, Makonnen E, *et al*. Long-term effect of efavirenz autoinduction on plasma/peripheral blood mononuclear cell drug exposure and CD4 count is influenced by UGT2B7 and CYP2B6 genotypes among HIV patients. J Antimicrob Chemother 2011.

[36] Yimer G, Amogne W, Habtewold A, *et al*. High plasma efavirenz level and CYP2B6*6 are associated with efavirenz-based HAART-induced liver injury in the treatment of naive HIV patients from Ethiopia: a prospective cohort study. Pharmacogenomics 2012; 12(6): 499-506.

[37] von Moltke LL, Greenblatt DJ, Granda BW, *et al*. Inhibition of Human Cytochrome P450 Isoforms by Nonnucleoside Reverse Transcriptase Inhibitors. J Clin Pharmacol 2001; 41(1): 85-91.

[38] Weiss J, Herzog M, Konig S, Storch CH, Ketabi-Kiyanvash N, Haefeli WE. Induction of multiple drug transporters by efavirenz. J Pharmacol Sci. 2009; 109(2): 242-50.

[39] Mouly S, Lown KS, Kornhauser D, *et al*. Hepatic but not intestinal CYP3A4 displays dose-dependent induction by efavirenz in humans. Clin Pharmacol Ther 2002; 72(1): 1-9.

[40] Whirl-Carrillo M, McDonagh EM, Hebert JM, *et al*. Pharmacogenomics knowledge for personalized medicine. Clin Pharmacol Ther 2012; 92(4): 414-7.

[41] Erickson DA, Mather G, Trager WF, Levy RH, Keirns JJ. Characterization of the *in vitro* biotransformation of the HIV-1 reverse transcriptase inhibitor nevirapine by human hepatic cytochromes P-450. Drug Metab Dispos 1999; 27(12): 1488-95.

[42] Riska P, Lamson M, MacGregor T, *et al*. Disposition and biotransformation of the antiretroviral drug nevirapine in humans. Drug Metab Dispos 1999; 27(8): 895-901.

[43] Wen B, Chen Y, Fitch WL. Metabolic activation of nevirapine in human liver microsomes: dehydrogenation and inactivation of cytochrome P450 3A4. Drug Metab Dispos 2009; 37(7): 1557-62.

[44] Faucette SR, Zhang TC, Moore R, *et al*. Relative activation of human pregnane X receptor *versus* constitutive androstane receptor defines distinct classes of CYP2B6 and CYP3A4 inducers. J Pharmacol Exp Ther 2007; 320(1): 72-80.

[45] Liptrott NJ, Pushpakom S, Wyen C, *et al*. Association of ABCC10 polymorphisms with nevirapine plasma concentrations in the German Competence Network for HIV/AIDS. Pharmacogenet Genomics 2012; 22(1): 10-9.

[46] Hopper-Borge E, Xu X, Shen T, Shi Z, Chen ZS, Kruh GD. Human multidrug resistance protein 7 (ABCC10) is a resistance factor for nucleoside analogues and epothilone B. Cancer Res 2009; 69(1): 178-84.

[47] Pushpakom SP, Liptrott NJ, Rodriguez-Novoa S, *et al*. Genetic variants of ABCC10, a novel tenofovir transporter, are associated with kidney tubular dysfunction. J Infect Dis 2011; 204(1): 145-53.

[48] Scholler-Gyure M, Kakuda TN, Raoof A, De Smedt G, Hoetelmans RM. Clinical pharmacokinetics and pharmacodynamics of etravirine. Clin Pharmacokinet 2009; 48(9): 561-74.

[49] James C, Preininger L, Sweet M. Rilpivirine: a second-generation nonnucleoside reverse transcriptase inhibitor. American journal of health-system pharmacy: AJHP 2012; 69(10): 857-61.

[50]   Dooley KE, Charles F, Andrade AS. Drug Interactions Involving Combination Antiretroviral Therapy and Other Anti-Infective Agents: Repercussions for Resource-Limited Countries. Journal of Infectious Diseases 2008; 198(7): 948-61.

[51]   Indiana University DoCP. P450 Drug Interaction Table: Abbreviated "Clinically Relevant" Table. Clin Pharmacol, 1001 W. 10th Street, WD W7123, Indianapolis, IN 46202 2011.

[52]   von Moltke LL, Greenblatt DJ, Grassi JM, *et al.* Protease inhibitors as inhibitors of human cytochromes P450: high risk associated with ritonavir. J Clin Pharmacol 1998; 38(2): 106-11.

[53]   Granfors MT, Wang JS, Kajosaari LI, Laitila J, Neuvonen PJ, Backman JT. Differential inhibition of cytochrome P450 3A4, 3A5 and 3A7 by five human immunodeficiency virus (HIV) protease inhibitors *in vitro*. Basic Clin Pharmacol Toxicol 2006; 98(1): 79-85.

[54]   Kirby BJ, Collier AC, Kharasch ED, Whittington D, Thummel KE, Unadkat JD. Complex drug interactions of HIV protease inhibitors 1: inactivation, induction, and inhibition of cytochrome P450 3A by ritonavir or nelfinavir. Drug Metab Dispos 2011; 39(6): 1070-8.

[55]   Josephson F. Drug–drug interactions in the treatment of HIV infection: focus on pharmacokinetic enhancement through CYP3A inhibition. J Intern Med 2010; 268(6): 530-9.

[56]   Database of Antiretroviral Drug Interactions: All Interactions with Nelfinavir (Viracept) [homepage on the Internet]. UCSF; 2014 [cited 23 February 2014]. Available from: http: //hivinsite.ucsf.edu/insite?page=ar-00-02&param=12&post=4#111/

[57]   Lu Y, Hendrix CW, Bumpus NN. Cytochrome P450 3A5 Plays a Prominent Role in the Oxidative Metabolism of the Anti-Human Immunodeficiency Virus Drug Maraviroc. Drug Metab Dispos 2012; 40(12): 2221-30.

[58]   AIDSinfo. Panel on Antiretroviral Guidelines for Adults and Adolescents. Guidelines for the use of antiretroviral agents in HIV-1-infected adults and adolescents. Department of Health and Human Services. AIDSinfo 2013.

[59]   WHO. New WHO guidelines recommend earlier treatment for people living with HIV, (accessed: 2013).

[60]   HIV and Viral Hepatitis [homepage on the Internet]. Updated: 2013. Available from: http: //www.cdc.gov/hiv/pdf/library_factsheets_HIV_and_viral_Hepatitis.pdf/

[61]   Larsen C, Pialoux G, Salmon D, *et al.* Prevalence of hepatitis C and hepatitis B infection in the HIV-infected population of France, 2004. Euro surveillance: bulletin Europeen sur les maladies transmissibles = European communicable disease bulletin 2008; 13(22).

[62]   Pereira K, Miranda AC, Baptista T, *et al.* Analysis of hepatitis non-treatment causes in a cohort of HCV and HCV/HIV infected patients. J Int AIDS Soc 2014; 17(4 Suppl 3): 19645.

[63]   Hartwell D, Jones J, Baxter L, Shepherd J. Peginterferon alfa and ribavirin for chronic hepatitis C in patients eligible for shortened treatment, re-treatment or in HCV/HIV co-infection: a systematic review and economic evaluation. Health technology assessment (Winchester, England) 2011; 15(17): i-xii, 1-210.

[64]   AIDSinfo. Guidelines for the Use of Antiretroviral Agents in HIV-1-Infected Adults and Adolescents. Drug Interactions between Nucleoside Reverse Transcriptase Inhibitors and Other Drugs (Including Antiretroviral Agents) AIDSinfo; 2013.

[65]   Solas C, Pambrun E, Winnock M, *et al.* Ribavirin and abacavir drug interaction in HIV-HCV coinfected patients: fact or fiction? AIDS (London, England) 2012; 26(17): 2193-9.

[66]   Amorosa VK, Slim J, Mounzer K, *et al.* The influence of abacavir and other antiretroviral agents on virological response to HCV therapy among antiretroviral-treated HIV-infected patients. Antiviral Ther 2010; 15(1): 91-9.

[67]   Pockros PJ. UpToDate: Direct-acting antivirals for the treatment of hepatitis C virus infection 2015. Available from: http://www.uptodate.com/contents/direct-acting-antivirals-for-the-treatment-of-hepatitis-c-virus-infection/

[68]   Beste LA, Green PK, Ioannou GN. Boceprevir and telaprevir-based regimens for the treatment of hepatitis C virus in HIV/HCV coinfected patients. Eur J Gastroenterol Hepatol 2015; 27(2): 123-9.

[69]   Coppola N, Martini S, Pisaturo M, Sagnelli C, Filippini P, Sagnelli E. Treatment of chronic hepatitis C in patients with HIV/HCV coinfection. World J Virol 2015; 4(1): 1-12.

[70]   Ghosal A, Yuan Y, Tong W, *et al*. Characterization of Human Liver Enzymes Involved in the Biotransformation of Boceprevir, a Hepatitis C Virus Protease Inhibitor. Drug Metab Dispos 2011; 39(3): 510-21.

[71]   Back D. Drug-drug interaction with new Hepatitis C drugs. Proceedings of the 5th Annual BHIVA conference on Management of HIV/Hepatitis Co-infection; 22 September 2012; One Great Gearge Street Conference Centre, London 2012.

[72]   Database of Antiretroviral Drug Interactions: Interactions between Antivirals (other) and Antiretrovirals [homepage on the Internet]. UCSF; 2014 [cited 30 April 2014]. Available from: http: //hivinsite.ucsf.edu/insite?page=ar-00-02&post=10&param=14.

[73]   Flanagan S, Crawford-Jones A, Orkin C. Simeprevir for the treatment of hepatitis C and HIV/hepatitis C co-infection. Expert Rev Clin Pharmacol 2014; 7(6): 691-704.

[74]   A SPECIAL MEETING REVIEW EDITION: Advances in the Treatment of Hepatitis C Virus Infection from The Liver Meeting 2013: Proceedings of the 64th Annual Meeting of the American Association for the Study of Liver Diseases. November 1-5, 2013; Washington DC. Gastroenterol Hepatol (N Y) 2014; 10(1 Suppl 1): 1-19.

[75]   Patel N, Nasiri M, Koroglu A, *et al*. Prevalence of Drug-Drug Interactions upon Addition of Simeprevir- or Sofosbuvir-Containing Treatment to Medication Profiles of Patients with HIV and Hepatitis C Coinfection. AIDS Res Hum Retroviruses 2015; 31(2): 189-97.

[76]   Younossi ZM, Stepanova M, Sulkowski M, *et al*. Sofosbuvir and Ribavirin for Treatment of Chronic Hepatitis C in Patients Coinfected With Hepatitis C Virus and HIV: The Impact on Patient-Reported Outcomes. J Infect Dis 2015.

[77]   Molina JM, Orkin C, Iser DM, *et al*. Sofosbuvir plus ribavirin for treatment of hepatitis C virus in patients co-infected with HIV (PHOTON-2): a multicentre, open-label, non-randomised, phase 3 study. Lancet 2015.

[78]   Ouwerkerk-Mahadevan S, Sekar V, Simion A, Peeters M, Beumont-Mauviel M. The Pharmacokinetic Interactions of the HCV Protease Inhibitor Simeprevir (TMC435) With HIV Antiretroviral Agents in Healthy Volunteers. In: Levin J, editor. IDSA Oct 17-21 2012; San Diego, UAS2012.

[79]   Database of Antiretroviral Drug Interactions: All Interactions with Simeprevir. [Internet]. 2013 [cited 27/03/2015].

[80]   Rusine J, Ondoa P, Asiimwe-Kateera B, *et al*. High seroprevalence of HBV and HCV infection in HIV-infected adults in Kigali, Rwanda. PloS one 2013; 8(5): e63303.

[81]   Imaoka T, Kusuhara H, Adachi M, Schuetz JD, Takeuchi K, Sugiyama Y. Functional involvement of multidrug resistance-associated protein 4 (MRP4/ABCC4) in the renal elimination of the antiviral drugs adefovir and tenofovir. Mol Pharmacol 2007; 71(2): 619-27.

[82]   Abu-Raddad LJ, Patnaik P, Kublin JG. Dual infection with HIV and malaria fuels the spread of both diseases in sub-Saharan Africa. Science 2006; 314(5805): 1603-6.

[83]   Korenromp EL, Williams BG, de Vlas SJ, *et al*. Malaria attributable to the HIV-1 epidemic, sub-Saharan Africa. Emerg Infect Dis 2005; 11(9): 1410-9.

[84]   UCSF. Malaria and HIV. 2006.

[85]   Birku Y, Mekonnen E, Bjorkman A, Wolday D. Delayed clearance of Plasmodium falciparum in patients with human immunodeficiency virus co-infection treated with artemisinin. Ethiop Med J 2002; 40 Suppl 1: 17-26.

[86]   Van Geertruyden JP, Mulenga M, Mwananyanda L, *et al*. HIV-1 immune suppression and antimalarial treatment outcome in Zambian adults with uncomplicated malaria. J Infect Dis 2006; 194(7): 917-25.

[87]   Achan J, Kakuru A, Ikilezi G, *et al*. Antiretroviral agents and prevention of malaria in HIV-infected Ugandan children. N Engl J Med 2012; 367(22): 2110-8.

[88]   Byakika-Kibwika P, Lamorde M, Mayito J, *et al.* Significant pharmacokinetic interactions between artemether/lumefantrine and efavirenz or nevirapine in HIV-infected Ugandan adults. J Antimicrob Chemother 2012; 67(9): 2213-21.

[89]   Guidelines for the Treatment of Malaria, (2010).

[90]   Byakika-Kibwika P, Lamorde M, Mayanja-Kizza H, Khoo S, Merry C, Van geertruyden J-P. Artemether-Lumefantrine Combination Therapy for Treatment of Uncomplicated Malaria: The Potential for Complex Interactions with Antiretroviral Drugs in HIV-Infected Individuals. Malar Res Treat 2011; 2011.

[91]   Mihara K, Svensson US, Tybring G, Hai TN, Bertilsson L, Ashton M. Stereospecific analysis of omeprazole supports artemisinin as a potent inducer of CYP2C19. Fundam Clin Pharmacol 1999; 13(6): 671-5.

[92]   Simonsson U, Jansson B, Hai T, Huong D, Tybring G, Ashton M. Artemisinin autoinduction is caused by involvement of cytochrome P450 2B6 but   not 2C9. Clin Pharmacol Therapy 2003; 74(1): 32-43.

[93]   Tan Bs. Population Pharmacokinetics of artesunate and its active metabolite dihydroartemisinin: Lowa University; 2009.

[94]   Burk O, Arnold KA, Nussler AK, Schaeffeler E, Efimova E, Avery BA. Antimalarial artemisinin drugs induce cytochrome P450 and MDR1 expression by activation of xenosensors pregnane X receptor and constitutive androstane receptor. Mol Pharmacol 2005; 67(6): 1954-65.

[95]   Elsherbiny DA, Asimus SA, Karlsson MO, Ashton M, Simonsson USH. A model based assessment of the CYP2B6 and CYP2C19 inductive properties by artemisinin antimalarials: Implications for combination regimens. Pharmacokinet Pharmacodyn 2008; 35(2): 203-17.

[96]   Parikh S, Gut J, Istvan E, Goldberg DE, Havlir DV, Rosenthal PJ. Antimalarial Activity of Human Immunodeficiency Virus Type 1 Protease Inhibitors. Antimicrob Agents Chemother 2005; 49(7): 2983-5.

[97]   Byakika-Kibwika P, Lamorde M, Okaba-Kayom V, *et al.* Lopinavir/ritonavir significantly influences pharmacokinetic exposure of artemether/lumefantrine in HIV-infected Ugandan adults. J Antimicrob Chemother 2012; 67(5): 1217-23.

[98]   Li XQ, Bjorkman A, Andersson TB, Ridderstrom M, Masimirembwa CM. Amodiaquine clearance and its metabolism to N-desethylamodiaquine is mediated by CYP2C8: a new high affinity and turnover enzyme-specific probe substrate. J Pharmacol Exp Ther 2002; 300(2): 399-407.

[99]   Preissner S, Kroll K, Dunkel M, *et al.* SuperCYP: a comprehensive database on Cytochrome P450 enzymes including a tool for analysis of CYP-drug interactions. Nucleic acids research. 2010; 38(Database issue): D237-43.

[100]   Fontaine F, de Sousa G, Burcham PC, Duchene P, Rahmani R. Role of cytochrome P450 3A in the metabolism of mefloquine in human and animal hepatocytes. Life sciences 2000; 66(22): 2193-212.

[101]   Lee TM, Huang L, Johnson MK, *et al. In vitro* metabolism of piperaquine is primarily mediated by CYP3A4. Xenobiotica 2012; 42(11): 1088-95.

[102]   Mirghani RA, Hellgren U, Bertilsson L, Gustafsson LL, Ericsson O. Metabolism and elimination of quinine in healthy volunteers. Eur J Clin Pharmacol 2003; 59(5-6): 423-7.

[103]   Allqvist A, Miura J, Bertilsson L, Mirghani RA. Inhibition of CYP3A4 and CYP3A5 catalyzed metabolism of alprazolam and quinine by ketoconazole as racemate and four different enantiomers. Eur J Clin Pharmacol 2007; 63(2): 173-9.

[104]   Mukonzo JK, Waako P, Ogwal-Okeng J, Gustafsson LL, Aklillu E. Genetic variations in ABCB1 and CYP3A5 as well as sex influence quinine disposition among Ugandans. Ther Drug Monit 32(3): 346-52.

[105]   Marcsisin S, Jin X, Bettger T, *et al.* CYP450 phenotyping and metabolite identification of quinine by accurate mass UPLC-MS analysis: a possible metabolic link to blackwater fever. Malaria journal 2013; 12(1): 214.

[106]   Bapiro TE, Andersson TB, Otter C, Hasler JA, Masimirembwa CM. Cytochrome P450 1A1/2 induction by antiparasitic drugs: dose-dependent increase in ethoxyresorufin O-deethylase

activity and mRNA caused by quinine, primaquine and albendazole in HepG2 cells. Eur J Clin Pharmacol 2002; 58(8): 537-42.

[107] Soyinka JO, Onyeji CO, Omoruyi SI, Owolabi AR, Sarma PV, Cook JM. Pharmacokinetic interactions between ritonavir and quinine in healthy volunteers following concurrent administration. Br J Clin Pharmacol 2010; 69(3): 262-70.

[108] Uriel A, Lewthwaite P. Malaria therapy in HIV: drug interactions between nevirapine and quinine. Int J STD AIDS 2011; 22(12): 768.

[109] Artesunate/Amodiaquine 100/270 mg tablet: WHOPAR part 6, MA058, (2011).

[110] Van Luin M, Van der Ende ME, Richter C, *et al*. Lower atovaquone/proguanil concentrations in patients taking efavirenz, lopinavir/ritonavir or atazanavir/ritonavir AIDS (London, England) 2010; 24 (8).

[111] Awewura KML, Kwamena WS, Fafa X, et al. Pharmacokinetics of Efavirenz when Co-administered with Rifampin in TB/HIV Co-infected Patients: Pharmacogenetic Effect of CYP2B6 Variation. J Clin Pharmacol 2008 2008; 48(9): 1032-40.

[112] Sousa M, Pozniak A, Boffito M. Pharmacokinetics and pharmacodynamics of drug interactions involving rifampicin, rifabutin and antimalarial drugs. J Antimicrob Chemother 2008; 62(5): 872-8.

[113] Court MFA, Greenblatt D, Duan S, Klein K, Zanger U, Kwara A. Identification of Isoniazid as a Potent Inhibitor of CYP2A6-mediated Efavirenz 7-hydroxylation in CYP2B6*6 Genotyped Human Liver Microsomes. Proceedings of Conference on Retrovirus and Opportunistic Infections; March 3-6th 2013; Georgia World Conference Centre: CROI; 2013.

[114] Wen X, Wang JS, Neuvonen PJ, Backman JT. Isoniazid is a mechanism-based inhibitor of cytochrome P450 1A2, 2A6, 2C19 and 3A4 isoforms in human liver microsomes. Eur J Clin Pharmacol 2002; 57(11): 799-804.

[115] Cohen K, Grant A, Dandara C, *et al*. Effect of rifampicin-based antitubercular therapy and the cytochrome P450 2B6 516G>T polymorphism on efavirenz concentrations in adults in South Africa. Antiviral Ther 2009; 14(5): 687-95.

[116] Ren Y, Nuttall JJ, Eley BS, *et al*. Effect of rifampicin on efavirenz pharmacokinetics in HIV-infected children with tuberculosis. J Acquir Immune Defic Syndr 2009; 50(5): 439-43.

[117] Klein UMZaK. Pharmacogenetics of cytochrome P450 2B6 (CYP2B6): advances on polymorphisms, mechanisms, and clinical relevance. Frontiers in Genetics | Pharmacogenetics and Pharmacogenomics. 2013; 4(24): 1-12.

[118] Eyakem AH. Pharmacokinetic and Pharmacogenetic aspects of drugdrug interactions between antiretroviral and antituberculosis drugs in Ethiopian patients: Implication for optimization of TB-HIV co-treatment. Stockholm: Karolinska Insitutet; 2013.

[119] Engels EA, Biggar RJ, Hall HI, *et al*. Cancer risk in people infected with human immunodeficiency virus in the United States. Int J Cancer 2008; 123(1): 187-94.

[120] Angeletti PC, Zhang L, Wood C. The viral etiology of AIDS-associated malignancies. Advances in pharmacology (San Diego, Calif) 2008; 56: 509-57.

[121] Mitsuyasu RT. Non--AIDS-defining malignancies in HIV. Topics in HIV medicine: a publication of the International AIDS Society, USA. 2008; 16(4): 117-21.

[122] Adjei A, Armah HB, Gbagbo F. Seroprevalence of HHV-8, CMV, and EBV among the general population in Ghana, West Africa. BMC infectious diseases 2008; 8: 111.

[123] Mwamba PM, Mwanda WO, Busakhala NW, Strother RM, Loehrer PJ, Remick SC. AIDS-Related Non-Hodgkin' s Lymphoma in Sub-Saharan Africa: Current Status and Realities of Therapeutic Approach. Lymphoma 2012; 2012: 9.

[124] Ulrickson M, Press OW, Casper C. Epidemiology, Diagnosis, and Treatment of HIV-Associated Non-Hodgkin Lymphoma in Resource-Limited Settings. Adv Hematol 2012; 2012: 7.

[125] Rudek MA, Flexner C, Ambinder RF. Use of antineoplastic agents in patients with cancer who have HIV/AIDS. Lancet 2011; 12(9): 905-12.

[126] Antoniou T. Potential Interactions between Antineoplastics and Antiretrovirals 2013. Available from: http: //www.hivclinic.ca/main/drugs_interact_files/Chemo-int.pdf/

[127] Baker SD, Hu S. Pharmacokinetic considerations for new targeted therapies. Clin Pharmacol Ther. 2009; 85(2): 208-11.

[128] Antoniou T, Tseng AL. Interactions between antiretrovirals and antineoplastic drug therapy. Clin Pharmacokinet 2005; 44(2): 111-45.

[129] Nallani SC, Goodwin B, Buckley AR, Buckley DJ, Desai PB. Differences in the induction of cytochrome P450 3A4 by taxane anticancer drugs, docetaxel and paclitaxel, assessed employing primary human hepatocytes. Cancer Chemother Pharmacol 2004; 54(3): 219-29.

Appendix: Summary of interations between ARVs and other commonly used agents

Group of drugs considered for interactions	Major enzyme/ transporter targets for the interaction	NRTI	NNRTI	PI	INSTI	Entry inhibitors
Other antiviral agents	Phosphrylation CYP3A4	Ribavirin interferes with phosphorylation of NRTI increasing virological failure Ribavirin-ddi combination is contraindicated due to increased intracellular levels of ddi and its toxicity Ribavirin increases hematological toxicity of AZT	Reduction in concentrations of boceprenavir/ teleprenavir during efavirenz co-administration	Bidirectional reduction in exposure during PI and boceprenavir/ teleprenavir co-administration	*Limited Data*	*Limited Data*
Antituberculosis treatment	CYP3A4/5, CYP2A6, CYP2B6, CYP1A2	Rifampicin induces uridyl glucuronyl transferases and increase AZT clearance	Rifampicin increases the metabolism of efavirenz and niverapine through induction of CYP3A4/5, CYP2A6, CYP2B6, CYP1A2,	Rifampicin increases the metabolism of efavirenz and niverapine through induction of CYP3A4/5, protease inhibitors	*Limited Data*	Rifampicin reduces bioavailability and exposure of Maraviroc.
Antimalarial agents	CYP2B6 CYP3A4/5 CYP2C8 Glucuronidation	*Limited Data*	Reduction in plasma levels of artmesinin, lumefantrine, efavirenz and niverapine due to CYP2B6, CYP2B6 and CYP3A4 induction Reduced exposure of quinine due to induction of CYP3A4 Efavirenz reduces plasma levels of atovaquine and proguanil following induction of glucuronidation and CYP2C8	Increased concetrations of ACTs due to CYP3A4 inhibition Reduced metabolism of quinine due to CYP3A4 inhibitions	*Limited Data*	Maraviroc may reduce levels of NNRTI/PI through CYP3A4 induction

Appendix contd….

| Anticancer agents | CYP3A4 CYP2C19 CYP2B6 | *Limited Data* | Clearance of vinca alkaloids may be increased due to CYP3A4 induction CYP2B6 induction by efavirenz or niverapine may lead to over production of the active metabolite of cyclophosphamide hence causing toxicity CYP2C19 Inhibition by etravrine may reduce production of active metabolite of cyclophosphamide Bleomycin may increace NNRTI concentrations following CY3A4 inhibition | Clearence of vinca alkaloids may be reduced due to CYP3A4 inhibition, hence increasing chances of toxicity Bleomycin may increace NNRTI concentrations following CY3A4 inhibition | CYP3A4 inibition by elvitegravir/ cobistat may reduce cyclophosphamide metabolism increasing its toxicity | *Limited Data* |

Frontiers in HIV Research, Vol. 1, 2015, 136-153

CHAPTER 8

Demographic Influence on the Evolution of Antiretroviral Therapy (ART)

Sarah Nanzigu[1,*], Moses R. Kamya[2] and Gene D. Morse[3,4]

[1]*Department of Pharmacology and Therapeutics, Makerere University College of Health Sciences, Uganda;* [2]*School of Medicine, Makerere University College of Health Sciences, Uganda;* [3]*Translational Pharmacology Research Core, NYS Center of Excellence in Bioinformatics and Life Sciences, USA and* [4]*School of Pharmacy and Pharmaceutical Sciences, University at Buffalo, USA*

Abstract: Access and well-modulated use of antiretroviral agents (ARVs) in North America dates as early as 1990 with the initial guidelines recommended zidovudine monotherapy, just 4 years after FDA approved the drug. Continued review of emerging data, led to the recommendation of highly active antiretroviral treatment (HAART) in 1998. Clear documentation of access and use of antiretroviral therapy (ART) in resource limited settings was first observed in 2002 after the World Health Organization (WHO) issued guidelines for resource limited settings, and included key ARVs into the WHO essential drug list. Delayed access to ART heavily impacted the initial control of the HIV epidemic in resource limited settings, but even with improved access to ART, differences in the management of HIV still exist; including timing for ART initiation and HIV/ART monitoring strategies. Access to key HIV/ART monitoring tools including viral load testing is limited in low resource settings, leading to gaps in HIV/ART management that may no longer be experienced in resource rich settings. Geographical variations in HIV sub-types and key co-infections further subject the control and management of HIV to demographic influence. Until now, resource availability and demographic differences are key determinants in treatment initiation and regimen selection, while variable access to ART and key monitoring tools possibly affect the HIV epidemic, making its control less effective in some settings.

Keywords: ART, Resource Settings, Resource Limited Settings, HIV, HIV/ART, HIV sub-types, ART Guidelines, HIV Co-treatment, ART Criteria, ART Timelines, ART Coverage.

INTRODUCTION

Life-saving antiretroviral therapy (ART) has been available for three decades since the development of the first antiretroviral drug, zidovudine, in 1985 [1-5].

Corresponding author Sarah Nanzigu: Department of Pharmacology and Therapeutics, Makerere University College of Health Sciences, Uganda; Tel: 256784843045, Fax: 256414532947; E-mails: snanzigu@yahoo.com; snanzigu@chs.mak.ac.ug

However, access and guidelines related to use of these agents differ with resource availability (Appendix **I**) [6-12]. It is now important to consider if variation in timelines related to the implementation of these therapies impact HIV/ART outcomes. This chapter summarizes the evolution of antiretroviral therapy (ART) since the beginning of the epidemic, in low and rich resource settings. Timelines in accessibility are based on guidelines that are followed by the different resource settings (Appendix **I**). This information is critically analyzed in line with the current data related to efficacy and/or toxicity of the available drugs, to reveal possible influences on the HIV epidemic. Geographical contributions to the HIV epidemic, including variation in HIV sub-types and the epidemiology of diseases that influence HIV virulence, and/or impact through co-treatments, are also examined.

Resource rich settings, including the United States, follow HIV/ART guidelines from the Department of Health and Human Services (DHHS) that are available at AIDSinfo.org [1, 7, 12]. The DHHS guidelines recommend use of individualized regimens that are selected based on virological efficacy, toxicity, pill burden, dosing frequency, drug-drug interaction potential, resistance testing, and co-morbid conditions [1]. On the other hand, resource limited settings follow the World Health Organization (WHO) guidelines developed largely for a public health approach in resource limited settings [8-11, 13-14]. Over time, differences have existed between the two resource settings with respect to accessibility, regimen selection, timing and monitoring of HIV/ART (Table **1**). These parameters affect HIV progression and transmissibility, hence, impacting the HIV epidemic in the two settings.

TIMELINES IN ART PROVISION AND ACCESS

Timelines in provision of ART have varied with resource availability. Following diagnosis of the first HIV/AIDS case, the first antiretroviral agents were developed and approved for use as monotherapy in the United States. This was the beginning of clinical research that would define the use of antiretroviral therapy. Evidence of access and well-modulated use of ART in resource limited settings was delayed for another decade, subjecting HIV infected persons to deteriorate without treatment, and making control of the epidemic difficult in the low resource settings (Table **1**). Prior to the initial guidelines for resource limited settings, there was no reliable evidence of guided use of ART in these settings where the HIV epidemic was worsening.

Table 1. The evolution in ART initiation criteria and key prognostic indicators: Differences in availability and content of guidelines has existed over time with reference to resource availability, and these differences could have impacted HIV/ART. ART coverage is based on WHO guidelines; prevalence is in adults while ADR refers to AIDS Related Deaths.

RESOURCE RICH SETTINGS Represented by USA		Year of Guideline	RESOURCE LIMITED SETTINGS Represented by sub Saharan Africa	
Key prognostic parameters	Criteria for ART initiation		Criteria for ART initiation	Key prognostic parameters
Prevalence <0.5% Unknown ART Coverage About 100,000 ARD	a. CD4 <200 b. CD4 200-500 +HIV symptoms c. AIDS complex	1993[6]	No guidelines	Prevalence =4% Unknown ART Coverage ≥500,000 ARD
Prevalence <1% Unknown ART Coverage About 50,000 ARD	a. CD4<500 b. VL>10,000 c. CD4 350-500 but VL<10,000; ART considered d. CD4>500, VL<10,000; minimal ART consideration	1998[7]	No guidelines	Prevalence= 5.8% Unknown ART Coverage ≥1,200,000 ARD
Prevalence <1% >25% ART coverage About 50,000 ARD	a. CD4<200 b. CD4 200-350; ART offered c. CD4>350, VL>550,000; ART considered d. Symptomatic HIV	2002 [8, 9]	a. CD4<200/mm3 or TLC <1200/mm3 b. WHO stages IIIb & IV	Prevalence= 5.9% 2 % ART coverage ≥1,500,000 ARD
Prevalence <1% 50% on ART 565,927 HIV deaths 56300 new infections	a. CD4<200 b. CD4 200-350; ART considered c. CD4>350 + VL>100,000; ART considered d. Symptomatic HIV	2006 [10, 11]	a. CD4≤200 b. WHO stage III + CD4 200-350; ART considered c. Pregnancy + WHO stage III + CD4<350 d. WHO stage IV	Prevalence=5.2% 23% ART coverage 2.1 million ARD 2.8 million new infections
Prevalence =0.5% 63% ART coverage 20,000 ARDs 580,000 new infections	a. CD4<350 b. CD4 350-500; ART considered c. CD4>500: ART considered d. HIVAN, active hepatitis B e. Pregnancy f. Symptomatic HIV	2010 [12, 13]	a. CD4≤350 b. WHO stage III-IV c. Pregnancy + CD4<350 or WHO stage III-IV d. Active TB or HBV	5% adult prevalence, 49% ART coverage 1.2 million ARD 1.9 million new infections
91 % on ART 20000 ARD 48,200 new infections	a. All HIV infected persons with priority at CD4 <500 b. Early HIV infection; ART offered	2013 [1, 14]	a. CD4≤500 b. All pregnant mothers c. All HIV serodiscordant persons in relations d. All children<5 years e. WHO stages III-IV	68 % on ART 1.2 million ARD 1.8 million new infections

The Effect of Varying Timelines in Provision and Access of ART

Impact on Progression of HIV Epidemic

The progression of the HIV epidemic is influenced by several factors including adult HIV prevalence and access to antiretroviral treatment. HIV infected persons are the source of new infections and hence, large numbers of untreated HIV infected persons translate into a higher mean community viral load leading to faster spread of the disease [15, 16]. On the other hand, use of antiretroviral therapy is associated with reduced viral load resulting in reduced risk of transmission [16]. Since the onset of HIV epidemic, ART coverage has been consistently lower in sub Saharan Africa compared to resource rich settings. Consequently, average viral load is 4-fold higher in sub Saharan Africa (highest in Southern and Eastern Africa) than in North America [15]. Untreated persons yielded a high average community VL over time, and this could have contributed to the persistent high HIV incidence in sub Saharan Africa, and Asia [15].

Despite the first antiretroviral agent being approved as early as 1986, the initial HIV/ART guidelines for resource limited settings were availed nearly two decades later, twice the time delay in resource rich settings (Table **1**). Although the initial DHHS guidelines were still undergoing extensive revisions, HIV treatment in resource rich settings, commenced as early as 1990, with zidovudine (ZDV) being recommended for post-exposure prophylaxis (PEP) [17]. By 1993 zidovudine, didanosine (ddI) and zalcitabine (ddC) were recommended for HIV treatment as monotherapy or in combination [6]. This early availability of zidovudine provided protection to persons exposed to HIV including children born to HIV infected mothers. The availability of guidelines and resources to access treatment early in the HIV epidemic could have greatly hampered the spread of the disease in North America; and assuming other factors remained constant, scarcity of resource influenced HIV control in Africa and Asia. None the less, monotherapy of zidovudine, zalcitabine and didanosine early in the epidemic, created a risk of resistance in settings where they were accessed rapidly [18].

The Impact on Disease Progression Among HIV Infected Persons

The WHO and UNAIDS developed key HIV progress indicators shown in Table **1**, and resource limited settings, particularly SSA, have shown poor indicators over time. AIDS related diseases and deaths, HIV prevalence, as well as infections in children, have all been higher in resource limited settings (Table **1**). At the onset of the epidemic, HIV prevalence was highest in SSA, while absence of guidelines in the early days, questions access and/or proper use of ART. The same data shows a progressive improvement in HIV progress indicators as ART coverage improved in both settings. On the other hand, the threshold for ART initiation remained low, only targeting patients with advanced infection, even after WHO included ART among essential drugs for RLS, [10-12]. Until 2006, ART in resource limited settings was commencing with CD4 <200 cells/mm^3, while resource rich settings have over time provided ART at CD4 ranging between 200-500 cells/ [10-12]. Key benefits of early treatment initiation on disease progression, including earlier suppression of viral replication, preservation of immune function and prolongation of disease-free survival were for a long time, missed in resource poor settings [23-25].

Despite the benefits of early ART, patients in resource rich settings might have had higher risks for problems related to prolonged ART including, adverse effects of these drugs on quality of life, reduced adherence due to inconveniencing regimens, risk of drug resistance during periods of suboptimal viral suppression, limitation of future treatment options following premature cycling of drugs and transmission of resistant virus. Nonetheless, disease progress was more controlled among HIV infected persons in well-resourced countries.

RESOURCE DIRECTED VARIABILITY IN CURRENT HIV/ART GUIDELINESS

Even with the improved access to ART, resource-related differences still exist with respect to regimen selection and HIV/ART monitoring (Table **2**). There are higher CD4 thresholds for ART provision in resource rich compared to resource limited settings, and while universal HIV/ART monitoring tools exist, availability and/or frequency of use differs in relation to resource availability, as detailed in Table **2**.

The Impact Created by Differences in Current Guidelines

The Effect from Differences in ART Initiation Criteria

The Department of Health and Human Services (DHHS) Panel on antiretroviral (ARV) guidelines for adults and adolescents recommends treating all HIV infected patients to reduce disease progression and transmission. The World Health Organization (WHO) recommends ART initiation at CD4<500 except for special populations including children, pregnant mothers, HIV positive patients in serodiscordant relationships and in cases of active TB or hepatitis co-infection. However, strength of the recommendation is at CD4<350.

❖ Early ART is associated with better treatment outcomes, and maintaining CD4 cell counts ≥500 is associated with a life expectancy equivalent to that of the general population [19]. This implies that HIV infected patients in resource rich settings could be having an extra benefit from early ART, and these are missed in low resource settings.

❖ Treatment before CD4 cell counts drop below 500 is associated with >90 % reduction in transmission [20, 21]. Delayed ART probably contributes to the higher HIV incidences in resource limited settings.

❖ Offering treatment during acute HIV infection (within 6 weeks of infection and before seroconversion) is associated with better treatment outcomes and its additional benefits include durable virological control, functional immune response during chronic HIV, reduced severity of the acute retroviral syndrome, preserved immune function and limited formation of HIV reservoirs [22-26]. There is currently no consideration for treating primary HIV in low resource settings, and hence, all cited benefits are foregone.

The Effect of Differences in Regimen Selection

Other than public directed ART in preference to individualized treatment in resource rich settings, specific difference in ART regimens exist between the two settings, and they include the following:

○ Delayed introduction of HIV protease inhibitors (PIs) into first line regimens for resource limited compared to resource rich settings (Table **2**). Research show PIs to have a higher genetic barrier to viral resistance compared to NNRTIs [27]. However, PIs are not yet included into first line regimens for resource limited settings. Over time, this might cause higher frequency of HIV resistance to less expensive and most accessible RTIs in resource limited settings. Resource-related storage requirements further reduce the number of PIs recommended for resource poor settings [28], while the requirement for viral load testing currently limits the use of rilpivirine.

○ Raltegravir (RAL) has a more durable virological response of up to 5 years when compared to efavirenz. It is however currently considered only for 3rd line regimens in resource limited settings [29-31].

Table 2. The 2013 HIV/ART guidelines: Differences between resource rich and limited settings.

Resource Rich Settings following DHHS Guidelines [1]	Focus of Guideline	Resource Limited Settings following WHO Guidelines [1]
a. All HIV infected persons although strength of recommendation differs by CD4 category; highest at CD4<350 and lowest at CD4 >500 b. To offer ART to persons with early HIV infection	Treatment Initiation	a. Asymptomatic; CD4≤500 but strongest recommendation at CD4<350 b. Pregnant and breast feeding mothers c. All HIV infected persons in serodiscordant relations d. All children<5 years e. WHO stages III-IV

First line regimens
a. NNRTI-Based Regimen: EFV/TDF/FTC
b. PI-Based: ATV-r + TDF+FTC or
    DRV-r + TDF+FTC
c. INSTI-Based: RAL + TDF+FTC
Alternatives:
NNRTI based: EFV + ABC/3TC
a. RPV/TDF/FTC   b. RPV + ABC/3TC
PI- based regimens
a. ATV/r + ABC+3TC
b. DRV/r + ABC+3TC
c. FPV/r + ABC+3TC/TDF/FTC
d. LPV/r + ABC+3TC/TDF/FTC
NSTI-Based Regimen
a. EVG+COBI+TDF+FTC in renal insufficiency
b. RAL + ABC+3TC
Rilpivirine (RPV) based ART if VL<100,000
	Recommended Antiretroviral drugs	**First line regimens**
		2NRTI + 1NNRTI
		  a. TDF +3TC/FTC + EFV (Preferred)
		  b. Alternative: AZT + 3TC + EFV
		  c. AZT + 3TC + NVP
		  d. TDF + 3TC / FTC + NVP
		
		Second lines
		2NRTI + PI-r
		a. AZT + 3TC + PI-r if TDF +3TC/FTC used in first line
		b. TDF +3TC/FTC + PI-r if AZT + 3TC used in first line
		
		Third lines
		Drugs with low risk of resistance
		Integrase inhibitors,
		Second generation NNRTI and PI

a. Entry into care b. Initiation/ modification of regimen c. 3-6 months before/ after initiating therapy d. 2-8 weeks into therapy to assess initial efficacy e. Treatment failure f. If clinically indicated	Timing of Viral Load testing	a. 6 Months after starting ART b. Every 12 on treatment c. Suspected treatment failure
a. Entry into care b. ART initiation c. 3-6 months before and after initiating ART d. 6-12 months in stable patients after starting ART e. Treatment failure f. Clinical indication	Timing for CD4 cell testing	a. Every 6-12 months before treatment b. ART initiation c. Every 6 months after starting ART d. At Treatment failure
a. Entry into care regardless of ART initiation b. Treatment initiation/ modification c. Treatment failure d. If clinically indicated	Timing for HIV resistance tests	Population level approach through surveillance of Development of HIV resistance. Otherwise use of warning indicators to development of resistance
When CCR5- Receptor antagonist use is considered	Co-receptor Tropism assay	Test/ guidelines not available

o   Maraviroc use is limited in RLS due to the need for CCR5 co-receptor tropism testing [32, 33].

The Impact Created by Differences in HIV/ART Monitoring

Differences have occurred in timelines related to the availability and application of HIV/ART monitoring tools, including; viral load testing and CD4 cell monitoring.

Effects of Varied Viral Load Testing

While frequent viral load testing was effected for individual patients in resource rich settings as early as 1998 [7], the test was not available in resource limited settings until 2006. Although full incorporation of the test into clinical care is currently considered for low resource settings, recommendations for viral load tests in RRS include establishing diagnosis when a syndrome consistent with acute HIV infection was present, making decisions related to treatment initiation, determination of initial ART efficacy 2-8 weeks after treatment initiation, assessment of durability of efficacy every 3-4 months, confirm treatment failure and whenever clinically indicated 1, 7, 8, 10, 12, 31, 35]. For a long time, WHO recommended use of viral load testing in resource limited settings to evaluate the emergence of HIV drug resistance at a population level, and the test is largely preserved for confirmation of resistance following clinical and or immunological failure [36].

The differences in access to viral load testing, may limit HIV/ART management in resource poor settings, eventually affecting treatment outcomes that are closely linked to this parameter. Viral load test results provide valuable information on ART efficacy and viral resistance, and delays in detecting suboptimal viral suppression has caused HIV treated patients to remain on failing regimens longer, increasing their risk of developing drug resistance[37, 38]. Some data have associated frequent viral load testing to reduced frequency of HIV drug resistance in a population [39, 40]. Despite conflicting data regarding the cost effectiveness for full incorporation of viral load monitoring into clinical care within resource limited settings, there is no doubt regarding the value added to clinical outcomes, as long as CD4 or viral load monitoring doesn't take precedence over ART expansion or regimen change [41-44]. Viral load monitoring leads to timely and complete detection of treatment failure, enabling timely switching to a second line

[45-50]. When compared to CD4 cell monitoring only, data from Southern Africa indicate an approximate four fold higher mortality in countries relying only on CD4 tests, compared to those where CD4 and viral load monitoring are combined [46]. While viral load testing in RLS has long been preserved to predict viral resistance after clinical or immunological failure, early testing during an ART regimen is very useful in providing information on initial efficacy and could predict disease progression and death to some extent [18, 51]. The test results also provide valuable information for regimen selection in non-treated HIV patients [52, 53]. These aspects are currently missed in low resource settings with limited access to the test.

Effects of Varied CD4 Cell Monitoring

CD4 cell testing is widely used for HIV/ART monitoring, however, until 2006, the test had limited accessibility in resource limited settings [9, 11, 54]. Prior to that, total T lymphocytes and clinical evaluation were the primary methods used to evaluate HIV/ART patients. Following improved access, the test is now recommended at diagnosis and, every 6 months, to decide on treatment initiation and continuation. The test was available in resource rich settings as early as 1993, with recommendations of its use at time of diagnosis, and every 3-6 months to decide on treatment initiation and continuation. Provided laboratory testing doesn't override the need for early treatment initiation or regimen change, immunological monitoring greatly adds clinical value, and this reduces the total health care expenditures related to hospitalization in cases where HIV-related problems are predictable from the test results [55, 56]

Effects of Varied HIV Resistance Testing

The 2010 and 2013 WHO guidelines recommend a population level surveillance of HIV drug resistance in RLS. On the contrary, HIV viral resistance tests were available for HIV infected individuals in resource rich settings as early as 2002. The recommendations for use in RRS include assessing baseline resistance prior to ART initiation, detecting suboptimal viral suppression and at the time of virological failure. In 2010, genotypic resistance testing was introduced for patients taking integrase inhibitors in RRS, but access to the test for clinical purposes is still very limited in RLS.

Data, including that available in the HIV drug resistance database, show significant viral resistance in different populations that would necessitate pre-treatment viral resistance testing [18, 37, 53, 57, 58]. Up to 12.9% resistance to NNRTI is estimated in Eastern Africa, 12% in Southern Africa, 15% in North America, and 10% for Canada, Europe and Asia [58]. Australia shows the highest HIV resistance prevalence of 23% [58]. Without pre-treatment HIV drug resistance testing, some patients are initiated on drugs with primary resistance mutations, therefore affecting treatment outcomes, and worsening the state of HIV drug resistance.

Chemokinine Co-receptor Tropism Assays

Following registration of maraviroc and findings of its limited activity on CXCR4-tropic virus, co-receptor tropism assays were introduced in 2010 for patients in whom use of CCR5- receptor antagonist was considered. However, the test is not yet available for clinical use in RLS. Although epidemiology of the CXCR4-tropic virus is not well documented, one study demonstrated 18% prevalence among patient samples from Canada [59]. On the other hand, up to 36% prevalence of CXCR4-coreceptor usage was detected among Ugandan HIV-positive patients with HIV1 subtype D [60]. HIV1 subtype D is the most prevalent subtype in Eastern Africa, and more aggressive compared to subtype B [61]. CXCR4 co-receptor usage is shown to increase with advancing HIV, and factors including low CD4 count and high viral load, are more prevalent in SSA and Asia. This suggests that Africa may be in much need for co-receptor tropism assay compared to other regions. However, the availability of the test is limited by resources.

INFLUENCE OF GENETICS ON HIV/ART IN THE TWO SETTINGS

Populations in both resource rich and poor setting differ in some genetic and disease characteristics, with implications on antiretroviral therapy. Some of these differences affect the efficacy of particular antiretroviral agents (Table **2**), while some agents have displayed racial differences in safety. Genetic diversity in HIV types and subtypes has delayed the development of a universal HIV vaccine, hence affecting control of the epidemic [62-66]. Further still, some differences in ART response measures have been linked to HIV diversity, although the clinical relevance of this is still being researched [67-70]. Table **3** details the effect of geographical and HIV diversity on HIV/ART.

Table 3(a). Differences in HIV virus subtypes and the possible implications on therapy.

Regional Distribution of HIV 1 main Subtypes	Observed Therapeutic Differences
N. America and Asia **B** is the predominant subtype	➤ HIV 1 subtype B showed reduced susceptibility to saquinavir and nelfinavir following L90M mutation [69]
South America **B** subtype is predominant C subtype occurs rarely	➤ HIV1 subtype G when compared to B was still susceptible to saquinavir, and had minimal reduction in susceptibility to nelfinavir after the L90M mutation [69] ➤ HIV 1 subtype B developed indinavir-related mutations M46I/L, I84V and V82A/F/T faster than subtype G [69]
Eastern Europe **A** is most predominant **B** is second predominant Others subtypes are still rare	➤ HIV 1 subtype A showed a 42.5-fold increased risk for the L210W mutation which confers resistance to NRTI [67] ➤ HIV 1 subtypes B and A were not observed to acquire the K20I mutation (confers resistance to PI) compared to 93-100% occurrence in subtype G [67]
Western Europe **C** is most predominant **B** is second predominant Other subtypes are still rare	➤ HIV 1 subtype C was shown to easily develop nelfinavir resistance *via* subtype specific pathways [68] ➤ Inhibition of HIV 1 subtype C by indinavir, ritonavir, saquinavir, and nelfinavir was 2– 4.5 fold weaker compared to subtype B [70] ➤ Inhibition of HIV 1 subtype A protease by indinavir, ritonavir, saquinavir, and nelfinavir was 2.5–7 fold weaker compared to subtype B [70]
Sub Saharan Africa **C** is most predominant **A & D** are second predominant B and CRF-AE still occur rarely	➤ HIV 1 subtype D was associated with fast disease progression and high rates of viral rebound [71, 72] ➤ CRF-AD polymorphism showed higher susceptibility to amprenavir and atazanavir [73] ➤ HIV 1Subtype G (prevalent in W. Africa) had an increased risk for A98G and V106I which confer resistance to NNRTI [67]

VARIATION IN HOST ENVIRONMENT AND IMPLICATIONS ON ART

Genetic differences in populations residing in the different resource settings have been reported, and they affect ART outcomes. Most of the reported effects relate to safety, and they include the following:

- Genetic polymorphisms related to efavirenz toxicity, specifically CYP2B6 polymorphisms are more prevalent in African and Papa New Guinea.

- Haplotype B (HLA-B*5701), which is associated with hypersensitivity to abacavir, is more common in Caucasians (5-8%) compared to Africans (3%).

HIV CO-INFECTION AND ITS POSSIBLE IMPLICATIONS

Table 3(b). Distribution of HIV Co-infections, and known implications on treatment.

HIV Co-infection	Resource Rich Settings	Resource Limited Settings	Key drug interactions
Tuberculosis HIV prevalence among TB patients in 2011 [74, 75]	5-19% in N. America 5-19% in Europe 0- 4 % in Canada 0- 4 % in Australia	>50% in SSA 20-49% in S. America 0-4 % in Asia	Rifampicin reduces plasma concentrations of the following drugs:- ➢ Efavirenz (NNRTI) ➢ Unboosted Protease Inhibitors ➢ Raltegravir (Integrase Inhibitor) ➢ Maraviroc (CCR5 antagonist) [76]
Malaria Reported malaria cases in 2010 (millions)	8.8 in USA 2.2 in Europe 14 in Western Pacific	110 in Africa 117 in S. E. Asia 12.9 in Eastern Mediterranean	NNRTI (Efavirenz and Niverapine) reduces plasma concentrations of artemether and lumefantrine leading to poor malaria treatment outcomes [77, 78] Delavirdine shows increased toxicity when combined with lumefantrine, artemether or halofantrine [79]
Viral Hepatitis C HCV prevalence in HIV patients	25% in US and France (≥80% for IDU) [80, 81]	1-5% [82-84]	Efavirenz (NNRTI) reduces the AUC of boceprevir and telaprevir
Viral Hepatitis B HBV prevalence in HIV patients	10% [80]	20-30% [85]	Cross resistance between the NRTI active against HBV (3TC, FTC, and active drugs like adefovir, delbivudine, entecavir) [85]

*HIV-1 estimated to increase malaria incidence by 1.3% in Africa (range 0.20 - 28%), highest in southern Africa [86]

CONFLICT OF INTEREST

The authors confirm that this chapter contents have no conflict of interest.

ACKNOWLEDGEMENTS

Declared none

REFERENCES

[1]   AIDSinfo. Panel on Antiretroviral Guidelines for Adults and Adolescents. Guidelines for the use of antiretroviral agents in HIV-1-infected adults and adolescents. Department of Health and Human Services. AIDSinfo 2013.

[2]   Clinical trial that led to FDA approval of zidovudine is published. Clinical pharmacy 1987; 6(10): 752.

[3]   Zidovudine (AZT). Lancet 1987; 1(8539): 957-8.

[4]   Zidovudine for AIDS. N Z Medical J 1987; 100(824): 331.

[5]   Hopkins S. Zidovudine treatment for AIDS. Nursing times 1987; 83(39): 64-5.

[6]   HIV Therapy Guidelines Issued [homepage on the Internet]. AIDinfo1993 [cited 06 November 2013]. Available from: http: //aidsinfo.nih.gov/news/65/hiv-therapy-guidelines-issued/

[7]   AIDSinfo. Report of the NIH Panel to Define Principles of Therapy of HIV Infection and Guidelines for the Use of Antiretroviral Agents in HIV-Infected Adults and Adolescents. Guidelines for the Use of Antiretroviral Agents in HIV-Infected adults and adolescents. U.S. DEPARTMENT OF HEALTH AND HUMAN SERVICES Centers for Disease Control and Prevention (CDC) Atlanta, Georgia 30333. AIDSinfo 1998.

[8]   AIDSinfo. Guidelines for the Use of Antiretroviral Agents in HIV-Infected Adults and Adolescents. AIDSinfo 2002.

[9]   Scaling up Antiretroviral Therapy in Resource-Limited Settings. Guidelines for a Public Health Approach. WHO 2002.

[10]   AIDSinfo. Guidelines for the Use of Antiretroviral Agents in HIV-1-Infected Adults and Adolescents. AIDSinfo 2006.

[11]   WHO. HIV/AIDS Programme. Strengthening health services to fight HIV/AIDS. Antiretroviral therapy for HIV infection in adults and adolescents: Recommendations for a public health approach. World Health Organization, 20 Avenue Appia, 1211 Geneva 27, Switzerland (tel.: +41 22 791 3264; fax: +41 22 791 4857: WHO Press 2006.

[12]   AIDSinfo. Panel on Antiretroviral Guidelines for Adults and Adolescents. Guidelines for the use of antiretroviral agents in HIV-1-infected adults and adolescents. Department of Health and Human Services. AIDSinfo 2009.

[13]   WHO. AntiretrovirAl therapy for hiv infection in Adults and Adolescents Recommendations for a public health approach. 2010.

[14]   New WHO guidelines recommend earlier treatment for people living with HIV. WHO 2013.

[15]   Abu-Raddad LJ, Barnabas RV, Janes H, *et al.* Have the explosive HIV epidemics in sub-Saharan Africa been driven by higher community viral load? AIDS 2013; 27(6): 981-9.

[16]   Das M, Chu PL, Santos GM, *et al.* Decreases in community viral load are accompanied by reductions in new HIV infections in San Francisco. PloS one 2010; 5(6): e11068.

[17]   Public Health Service Statement on Management of Occupational Exposure to Human Immunodeficiency Virus, Including Considerations Regarding Zidovudine Postexposure Use [Internet]. AIDSinfo 1990 [cited 07 November 2013]. Available from: http://aidsinfo.nih.gov/news/113/public-health-service-statement-on-management-of-occupational-exposure-to-human-immunodeficiency-virus-including-considerations-regarding-zidovudine-postexposure-use/

[18]   Brun-Vezinet F, Boucher C, Loveday C, *et al.* HIV-1 viral load, phenotype, and resistance in a subset of drug-naive participants from the Delta trial. The National Virology Groups. Delta Virology Working Group and Coordinating Committee. Lancet 1997; 350(9083): 983-90.

[19]   Rodger AJ, Lodwick R, Mauro S, *et al.* Mortality in well controlled HIV in the continuous antiretroviral therapy arms of the SMART and ESPRIT trials compared with the general population. AIDS 2013; 27(6): 973-9.

[20]   Anglemyer A, Rutherford GW, Baggaley RC, *et al.* Antiretroviral therapy for prevention of HIV transmission in HIV-discordant couples. Cochrane Database Syst Rev 2011(8): CD009153.

[21]   Cohen MS, McCauley M, Gamble TR. HIV treatment as prevention and HPTN 052. Curr Opin HIV AIDS. 2012; 7(2): 99-105.

[22]   Bell SK, Little SJ, Rosenberg ES. Clinical management of acute HIV infection: best practice remains unknown. J Infect Dis 2010; 202 Suppl 2: S278-88.

[23]   Jain V, Hartogensis W, Bacchetti P, *et al.*, editors. Antiretroviral Therapy Initiation during Acute/Early HIV Infection *vs.* Later ART Initiation is Associated with Improved Immunologic and Virologic Parameters during Suppressive ART. Proceedings of the 18th CROI (Conference on Retroviruses and Opportunistic Infections); February 27 - March 2, 2011; Boston, MA.

[24]   Lisziewicz J, Rosenberg E, Lieberman J, *et al.* Control of HIV despite the Discontinuation of Antiretroviral Therapy. N Engl J Med 1999; 340(21).

[25]   Oxenius A, Price DA, Easterbrook PJ, *et al.* Early highly active antiretroviral therapy for acute HIV-1 infection preserves immune function of CD8+ and CD4+ T lymphocytes. Proceedings of the National Academy of Sciences. 2000; 97(7): 3382-7.

[26]   Rosenberg ES, Altfeld M, Poon SH, *et al.* Immune control of HIV-1 after early treatment of acute infection. Nature 2000; 407(6803): 523-6.

[27]   Luber AD. Genetic barriers to resistance and impact on clinical response. MedGenMed: Medscape general medicine 2005; 7(3): 69.

[28]   AIDSinfo. Guidelines for the Use of Antiretroviral Agents in HIV-1-Infected Adults and Adolescents. Appendix B: Drug Characteristics: AIDSinfo 2013.

[29]   DeJesus E, Rockstroh JK, Lennox JL, *et al.* Efficacy of raltegravir *versus* efavirenz when combined with tenofovir/emtricitabine in treatment-naive HIV-1-infected patients: week-192 overall and subgroup analyses from STARTMRK. HIV clinical trials 2012; 13(4): 228-32.

[30]   Eron JJ, Cooper DA, Steigbigel RT, *et al.* Efficacy and safety of raltegravir for treatment of HIV for 5 years in the BENCHMRK studies: final results of two randomised, placebo-controlled trials. The Lancet infectious diseases 2013; 13(7): 587-96.

[31]   Rockstroh JK, DeJesus E, Lennox JL, *et al.* Durable efficacy and safety of raltegravir *versus* efavirenz when combined with tenofovir/emtricitabine in treatment-naive HIV-1-infected patients: final 5-year results from STARTMRK. J AIDS 2013; 63(1): 77-85.

[32]   Westby M. Resistance to CCR5 antagonists. Curr Opin HIV AIDS 2007; 2(2): 137-44.

[33]   Westby M, van der Ryst E. CCR5 antagonists: host-targeted antivirals for the treatment of HIV infection. Antivir Chem Chemother 2005; 16(6): 339-54.

[34]   AIDSinfo. Guidelines for the Use of Antiretroviral Agents in HIV-1-Infected Adults and Adolescents. AIDSinfo 2003.

[35]   AIDSinfo. Panel on Antiretroviral Guidelines for Adults and Adolescents. Guidelines for the use of antiretroviral agents in HIV-1-infected adults and adolescents. Department of Health and   Human Services 2012.

[36]   HIV/AIDS Programme. Strengthening health services to fight HIV/AIDS. Antiretroviral therapy for HIV infections in adults and adolescents: Recommendations for a public health approach- WHO 2006.

[37]   Adje-Toure CA, Cheingsong R, Garcia-Lerma JG, *et al.* Antiretroviral therapy in HIV-2-infected patients: changes in plasma viral load, CD4+ cell counts, and drug resistance profiles of patients treated in Abidjan, Cote d'Ivoire. Aids 2003; 17 Suppl 3: S49-54.

[38]   Germanaud D, Derache A, Traore M, *et al.* Level of viral load and antiretroviral resistance after 6 months of non-nucleoside reverse transcriptase inhibitor first-line treatment in HIV-1-infected children in Mali. J Antimicrob Chemother 2010; 65(1): 118-24.

[39]   Assoumou L, Descamps D, Yerly S, *et al.* Prevalence of HIV-1 drug resistance in treated patients with viral load >50 copies/mL in 2009: a French nationwide study. J Antimicrob Chemother 2013; 68(6): 1400-5.

[40]   Charest H, Doualla-Bell F, Cantin R, *et al.* A significant reduction in the frequency of HIV-1 drug resistance in Quebec from 2001 to 2011 is associated with a decrease in the monitored viral load. PloS one 2014; 9(10): e109420.

[41]   Mermin J, Ekwaru JP, Were W, *et al.* Utility of routine viral load, CD4 cell count, and clinical monitoring among adults with HIV receiving antiretroviral therapy in Uganda: randomised trial. BMJ 2011; 343: d6792.

[42]   Phillips AN, Pillay D, Miners AH, *et al.* Outcomes from monitoring of patients on antiretroviral therapy in resource-limited settings with viral load, CD4 cell count, or clinical observation alone: a computer simulation model. Lancet 2008; 371(9622): 1443-51.

[43]   Schneider K, Puthanakit T, Kerr S, *et al.* Economic evaluation of monitoring virologic responses to antiretroviral therapy in HIV-infected children in resource-limited settings. AIDS 2011; 25(9): 1143-51.

[44]   Scott Braithwaite R, Nucifora KA, Toohey C, *et al.* How do different eligibility guidelines for antiretroviral therapy affect the cost-effectiveness of routine viral load testing in sub-Saharan Africa? AIDS 2014; 28 Suppl 1: S73-83.

[45]   Davies MA, Boulle A, Technau K, *et al.* The role of targeted viral load testing in diagnosing virological failure in children on antiretroviral therapy with immunological failure. Trop Med Int Health 2012; 17(11): 1386-90.

[46]   Estill J, Egger M, Johnson LF, *et al.* Monitoring of antiretroviral therapy and mortality in HIV programmes in Malawi, South Africa and Zambia: mathematical modelling study. PloS one 2013; 8(2): e57611.

[47]   Keiser O, MacPhail P, Boulle A, *et al.* Accuracy of WHO CD4 cell count criteria for virological failure of antiretroviral therapy. Tropical medicine & international health: TM & IH 2009; 14(10): 1220-5.

[48]   Keiser O, Tweya H, Braitstein P, *et al.* Mortality after failure of antiretroviral therapy in sub-Saharan Africa. Tropical medicine & international health: TM & IH 2010; 15(2): 251-8.

[49]   Salazar-Vizcaya L, Keiser O, Karl T, *et al.* Viral load *versus* CD4 (+) monitoring and 5-year outcomes of antiretroviral therapy in HIV-positive children in Southern Africa: a cohort-based modelling study. AIDS 2014; 28(16): 2451-60.

[50]   Sigaloff KC, Hamers RL, Wallis CL, *et al.* Unnecessary antiretroviral treatment switches and accumulation of HIV resistance mutations; two arguments for viral load monitoring in Africa. J AIDS 2011; 58(1): 23-31.

[51]   Hughes MD, Johnson VA, Hirsch MS, *et al.* Monitoring plasma HIV-1 RNA levels in addition to CD4+ lymphocyte count improves assessment of antiretroviral therapeutic response. ACTG 241 Protocol Virology Substudy Team. Ann Intern Med 1997; 126(12): 929-38.

[52]   Chin BS, Choi J, Nam JG, *et al.* Inverse relationship between viral load and genotypic resistance mutations in Korean patients with primary HIV type 1 infections. AIDS Res Hum Retroviruses 2006; 22(11): 1142-7.

[53]   Harrison L, Castro H, Cane P, *et al.* The effect of transmitted HIV-1 drug resistance on pre-therapy viral load. AIDS 2010; 24(12): 1917-22.

[54]   WHO. Scaling up antiretroviral therapy in Resource-limited settings: Treatment guidelines for a public health approach. Geneva, Switzerland: WHO 2003.

[55]   Bendavid E, Young SD, Katzenstein DA, *et al.* Cost-effectiveness of HIV monitoring strategies in resource-limited settings: a southern African analysis. Arch Intern Med 2008; 168(17): 1910-8.

[56]   Team DT, Mugyenyi P, Walker AS, *et al.* Routine *versus* clinically driven laboratory monitoring of HIV antiretroviral therapy in Africa (DART): a randomised non-inferiority trial. Lancet 2010; 375(9709): 123-31.

[57]   Ndembi N, Goodall RL, Dunn DT, *et al.* Viral rebound and emergence of drug resistance in the absence of viral load testing: a randomized comparison between zidovudine-lamivudine plus Nevirapine and zidovudine-lamivudine plus Abacavir. J Infect Dis 2010; 201(1): 106-13.

[58]   HIV-1 Drug Resistance in ARV-naive Populations [Internet]. 2013 [cited 11 November 2013]. Available from: http://hivdb.stanford.edu/surveillance/map/.

[59]   Brumme ZL, Goodrich J, Mayer HB, *et al.* Molecular and clinical epidemiology of CXCR4-using HIV-1 in a large population of antiretroviral-naive individuals. J Infect Dis 2005; 192(3): 466-74.

[60]   Huang W, Eshleman SH, Toma J, *et al.* Coreceptor tropism in human immunodeficiency virus type 1 subtype D: high prevalence of CXCR4 tropism and heterogeneous composition of viral populations. J Virol 2007; 81(15): 7885-93.

[61]   Baeten JM, Chohan B, Lavreys L, *et al.* HIV-1 subtype D infection is associated with faster disease progression than subtype A in spite of similar plasma HIV-1 loads. J Infect Dis 2007; 195(8): 1177-80.

[62]   Excler JL, Tomaras GD, Russell ND. Novel directions in HIV-1 vaccines revealed from clinical trials. Curr Opin HIV AIDS 2013; 8(5): 421-31.

[63]   KE. S, DH. B. A global approach to HIV-1 vaccine development. Immunological reviews 2013; 254(1): 295-304.

[64]   Pantophlet R. Antibody epitope exposure and neutralization of HIV-1. Curr Pharm Des 2010; 16(33): 3729-43.

[65]   Pantophlet R, Burton DR. GP120: target for neutralizing HIV-1 antibodies. Annu Rev Immunol 2006; 24: 739-69.

[66]   Prentice HA, Ehrenberg PK, Baldwin KM, *et al.* HLA class I, KIR, and genome-wide SNP diversity in the RV144 Thai phase 3 HIV vaccine clinical trial. Immunogenetics 2014; 66(5): 299-310.

[67]   Chaplin B, Eisen G, Idoko J, *et al.* Impact of HIV type 1 subtype on drug resistance mutations in Nigerian patients failing first-line therapy. AIDS Res Hum Retroviruses 2011; 27(1): 71-80.

[68]   Doualla-Bell F, Avalos A, Gaolathe T, *et al.* Impact of human immunodeficiency virus type 1 subtype C on drug resistance mutations in patients from Botswana failing a nelfinavir-containing regimen. Antimicrob Agents Chemother 2006; 50(6): 2210-3.

[69]   Santos AF, Abecasis AB, Vandamme AM, *et al*. Discordant genotypic interpretation and phenotypic role of protease mutations in HIV-1 subtypes B and G. J Antimicrob Chemother 2009; 63(3): 593-9.
[70]   Velazquez-Campoy A, Todd MJ, Vega S, *et al*. Catalytic efficiency and vitality of HIV-1 proteases from African viral subtypes. Proceedings of the National Academy of Sciences; 2001; 98(11): 6062-7.
[71]   Easterbrook PJ, Smith M, Mullen J, *et al*. Impact of HIV-1 viral subtype on disease progression and response to antiretroviral therapy. J Int AIDS Soc 2010; 13: 4.
[72]   Martinez-Cajas JL, Pant-Pai N, Klein MB, *et al*. Role of genetic diversity amongst HIV-1 non-B subtypes in drug resistance: a systematic review of virologic and biochemical evidence. AIDS reviews 2008; 10(4): 212-23.
[73]   Santos AF, Tebit DM, Lalonde MS, *et al*. Effect of natural polymorphisms in the HIV-1 CRF02_AG protease on protease inhibitor hypersusceptibility. Antimicrob Agents Chemother 2012; 56(5): 2719-25.
[74]   AIDS.Gov. Tuberculosis and HIV 2013 [14 November 2013]. Available from: http: //www.aids.gov/hiv-aids-basics/staying-healthy-with-hiv-aids/potential-related-health-problems/tuberculosis/.
[75]   Tuberculosis and HIV Data: Estimated HIV prevalence among TB cases, 2011 [homepage on the Internet]. WHO; 2011. Available from: http: //www.who.int/hiv/topics/tb/data/en/.
[76]   Tuberculosis and HIV [homepage on the Internet]. UCSF; 2013. Available from: http: //hivinsite.ucsf.edu/InSite?page=kb-05-01-06#S2X/
[77]   Achan J, Kakuru A, Ikilezi G, *et al*. Antiretroviral agents and prevention of malaria in HIV-infected Ugandan children. N Engl J Med 2012; 367(22): 2110-8.
[78]   Byakika-Kibwika P, Lamorde M, Mayito J, *et al*. Significant pharmacokinetic interactions between artemether/lumefantrine and efavirenz or nevirapine in HIV-infected Ugandan adults. J Antimicrob Chemother 2012; 67(9): 2213-21.
[79]   UCSF. Malaria and HIV 2006.
[80]   HIV and Viral Hepatitis [homepage on the Internet]. CDC; 2013. Available from: http: //www.cdc.gov/hiv/pdf/library_factsheets_HIV_and_viral_Hepatitis.pdf.
[81]   Larsen C, Pialoux G, Salmon D, *et al*. Prevalence of hepatitis C and hepatitis B infection in the HIV-infected population of France, 2004. Euro surveillance: bulletin Europeen sur les maladies transmissibles = European communicable disease bulletin 2008; 13(22).
[82]   Kapembwa KC, Goldman JD, Lakhi S, *et al*. HIV, Hepatitis B, and Hepatitis C in Zambia. J Global Infect Dis 2011; 3(3): 269-74.
[83]   Rusine J, Ondoa P, Asiimwe-Kateera B, *et al*. High seroprevalence of HBV and HCV infection in HIV-infected adults in Kigali, Rwanda. PloS one 2013; 8(5): e63303.
[84]   Walusansa V, Kagimu M. Screening for hepatitis C among HIV positive patients at Mulago hospital in Uganda. Afri Health Sci 2009; 9(3): 143-6.
[85]   Hepatitis B and HIV con-infection [Internet]. 2010. Available from: http: //hivinsite.ucsf.edu/InSite?page=kb-05-03-04#S1X.
[86]   Korenromp EL, Williams BG, de Vlas SJ, *et al*. Malaria attributable to the HIV-1 epidemic, sub-Saharan Africa. Emerg Infect Dis 2005; 11(9): 1410-9.

Appendix I: Table showing timelines for availability and/or accessibility of different antiretroviral agents basing on guidelines applied in either resource limited and resource rich settings

Generic Name	Year of FDA Approval	Year of Initial Recommendation by DDHS	Year of Initial Recommendation by WHO for Resource Limited Settings
Nucleoside Reverse Transcriptase Inhibitors (NRTIs)			
Emtricitabine (FTC)	2003	2004	2006
Tenofovir disoproxil fumarate (TDF)	2001	2004	2003
Enteric coated didanosine (ddI EC)	2000		
Abacavir sulfate (ABC)	1998	1998	2002
Lamivudine (3TC)	1995	1998	2002
Stavudine (d4T)	1994	1998	2002
Zalcitabine (dideoxycytidine,ddC) No longer marketed	1992	1993	
Didanosine (ddI)	1991	1993	2002
Zidovudine (AZT)	1987	1990	2002
Non-nucleoside Reverse Transcriptase Inhibitors (NNRTIs)			
Rilpivirine	2011	2013	
Etravirine	2008	2008	
Efavirenz (EFV)	1998	1998	2002, WHO expanded use to first trimester and children <3yrs in 2013
Delavirdine (DLV)	1997		
sNevirapine Immediate release (NVP)	1996	1998	2002
Nevirapine extended release	2011		
Rilpivirine if VL<100,000		2013	
Protease Inhibitors (PIs)			
Amprenavir (APV) (no longer marketed)	1999		
Tipranavir (TPV)	2005		
Indinavir (IDV)	1996	1998	2002
Saquinavir mesylate (SQV)	1995	1998	2002
Lopinavir + Ritonavir (LPV/RTV)	2000	1998	2002
Fosamprenavir Calcium(FOS-APV)	2003		

Appendix I: contd…

Ritonavir (RTV)	1996	1998	2002
Darunavir	2006		
Atazanavir sulphate (ATV)	2003		2010
Atazanavir + Ritonavir			2010
Nelfinavir mesylate (NFV)	1997	1998	2002
Fusion Inhibitors			
Enfuvirtide (T-20)	2003		

Entry Inhibitors- CCR5 Co-receptor Antagonists

Maraviroc	2007		

HIV Integrase Strand Inhibitors

Raltegravir	2007		
Elvitegravir	2012		
Dolutegravir	2013		

Others

Cobicistat (Booster)		2013	

Subject Index